The Periodontic-Endodontic Interface

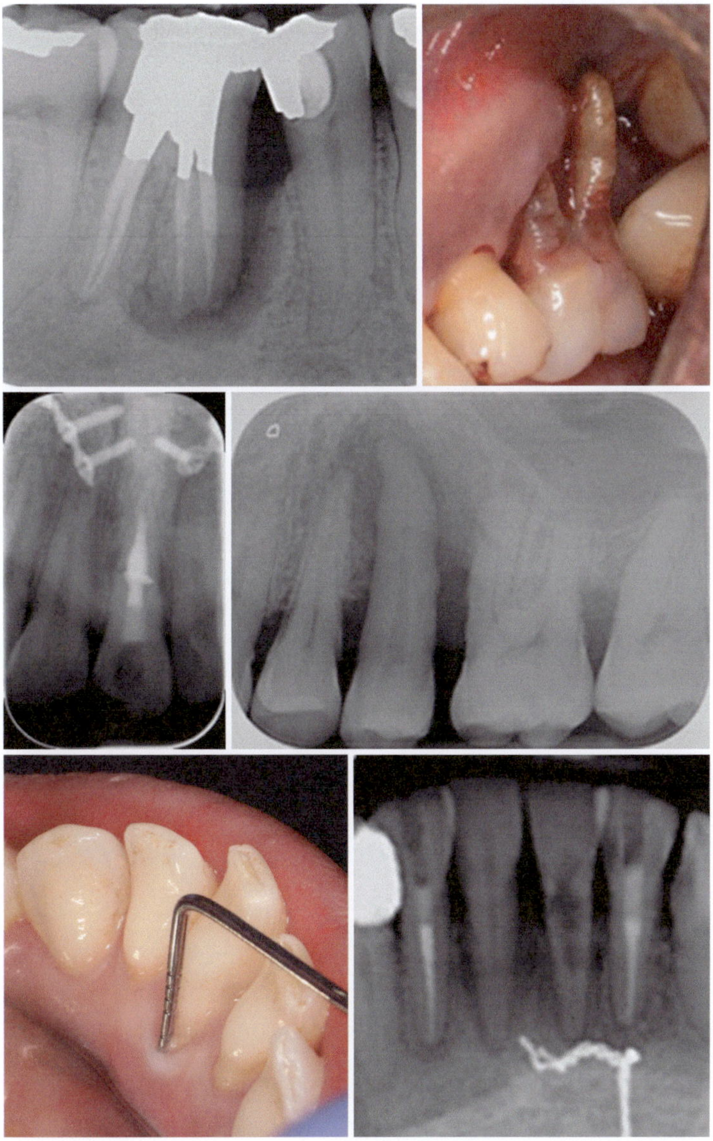

Shiyana Eliyas

The Periodontic-Endodontic Interface

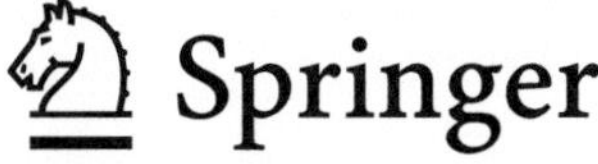
Springer

Shiyana Eliyas, BDS, MFDS, MRD, FDS, PhD
Department of Restorative Dentistry
St George's Hospitals NHS Foundation Trust
London, UK

ISBN 978-3-031-49939-5   ISBN 978-3-031-49937-1   (eBook)
https://doi.org/10.1007/978-3-031-49937-1

This Springer imprint is published by the registered company Springer Nature Switzerland AG
The registered company address is: Gewerbestrasse 11, 6330 Cham, Switzerland

Paper in this product is recyclable.

I dedicate this book to my Mother, Fawziya, and Stepfather, Suhail, who helped me to learn to read and write in English when I first arrived in England. They spent endless hours giving my siblings and I extra homework, spelling tests and marking our various attempts at re-writing the chapters of our favourite books.

Preface

The periodontium consists of the external supporting soft and hard tissues of the tooth. The root canal system houses the internal blood supply to the vital pulp-dentine complex of the tooth (the endodontium) that makes the tooth a living structure. Both the periodontium and the endodontium are at risk of developing disease separately and can be treated separately to varying degrees of success; however, when they present together, combined periodontal and endodontic lesions (perio-endo lesions) are a quandary in treatment. Perio-endo lesions are considered a prognostic indicator for poor outcomes of treatment, usually determined by the outcome of the periodontal treatment. The diagnosis is of importance because those lesions that appear to be perio-endo lesions but are solely of endodontic origin will heal with endodontic intervention, whereas periodontal disease with irreversible endodontic manifestations and true perio-endo lesions will require both periodontal and endodontic treatment, and be reliant on the patient's compliance of good oral hygiene with modification of aetiological factors to achieve success. The aim of this book is to lead the reader to a better understanding of the periodontic-endodontic interface, the aetiology and diagnosis of perio-endo lesions, and therefore, management of such lesions.

London, UK   Dr. Shiyana Eliyas

Text

This book equips dental care providers with a thorough understanding of the Periodontic-Endodontic Interface. It discusses embryonic development of the tooth, oral health and pathology, as well as the diagnosis and management of periodontal disease and endodontic disease, occurring both separately and together. Evidence-based information is given on periodontic and endodontic pathogens, lesions and infections with various forms of their manifestations. The clear and easy-to-read text is complemented by numerous high-quality photographs and tables that assist understanding and help with the identification of management solutions. The book is a valuable resource for all dental practitioners with an interest in endodontics, periodontics, restorative dentistry, and for higher-level students.

USPs

Discusses periodontal and endodontic disease, occurring both separately and together
Includes clinical cases to illustrate practical tips
Gives evidence-based information on lesions, infections and oral health

SEO MetaData

This book equips dental care providers with a thorough understanding of the Periodontic-Endodontic Interface.

Acknowledgements

Thank you to those who supplied images for this book:

- Image 2 of Page I—picture courtesy of Miss Rhianna Clarke
- Image 5 of Page I—picture courtesy of Mr. Alexander Buzar-Jomehri
- Figure 5.4—pictures courtesy of Mr. Vithurran Vijayenthiran
- Figure 5.5—case and pictures courtesy of Mr. Peter Briggs
- Figure 8.6—case courtesy of Mr. Nalin Dhamecha

With thanks to Peter Briggs for reading the early draft, and my mother for all of her guidance, help and proof reading.

Thank you also to all those who contributed to my training over the years. I have tried to include the 'golden nuggets' in this book.

Competing Interests

There are no competing interests in relation to the context of this book.

Contents

About the Author

Dr. Shiyana Eliyas, BDS, MFDS, PGCert (Higher Ed), MRD, FDS (Rest Dent), PhD GDC No. 81114. Registered with the GDC as a specialist in Restorative Dentistry, Endodontics, Periodontics and Prosthodontics.

Dr. Eliyas is a Consultant in Restorative Dentistry at St George's University Hospital Foundation Trust. Following graduation from King's College London in 2002, she gained experience in a variety of environments including teaching hospitals, district general hospitals, as well as National Health and Private practice. Dr. Eliyas has undertaken Specialty Training in Restorative Dentistry at Sheffield Teaching Hospitals NHS Foundation Trust and completed a Head and Neck Oral Rehabilitation Fellowship in Manchester and Liverpool Dental Hospitals. She achieved a Doctorate on the feasibility of measuring the quality of post-graduate education in endodontics in primary care using outcomes of endodontic treatment. She has published widely and enjoys teaching and research.

Dr. Eliyas clinical interests lies in the management of complex restorative dental problems including endodontic, periodontal and prosthetic issues as well as the management of peri-implant disease. Her current position includes managing complex restorative problems in high priority patients (head and neck cancer, those with dento-alveolar trauma and those with dental developmental disorders). She is currently the President of the British Society of Prosthodontics.

Introduction

1

Abstract

This chapter gives an introduction to the periodontic-endodontic (perio-endo) interface. It describes the importance of saving teeth and compares the alternative replacement options. The learning objectives of this book are set out at the end of this first chapter.

Introduction

The tissues of the periodontium and endodontium communicate with each other embryologically for their development, anatomically once the tooth has erupted into the oral cavity as part of their normal function during health, as well as pathologically when disease develops. It has been said that 50% of tooth mortality might show periodontal and pulpal pathology (Chen et al. 1997). That coupled with patients living for longer, as well as the recent increasing awareness and motivation of patients to keep their teeth for longer, is likely to mean that the number of teeth needing periodontal and endodontic treatment in the population is vast. Both periodontal and endodontic structures of a tooth are closely linked and the handling of one structure may affect the other.

Generally the periodontic-restorative interface is in the region of the gingival margin of the tooth. The patients and clinicians influence on this area is related to the development of caries and marginal bone loss. The placement of the restoration itself may harm the gingival tissues (trauma from the removal of caries, the placement of rubber dam, matrix bands and wooden wedges, for example) and the material placed may continue to irritate the periodontal tissues long after completion of the procedure. Occasionally there is development of cervical or invasive external resorption, which may also instigate the placement of restorations in this region;

© The Author(s), under exclusive license to Springer Nature Switzerland AG 2024
S. Eliyas, *The Periodontic-Endodontic Interface*,
https://doi.org/10.1007/978-3-031-49937-1_1

again the method of restoration (surgical or non-surgical) and material used will impact the reaction of the periodontal tissues, with or without a pathological response.

A 26-year longitudinal study compared periodontal outcomes of teeth with and without restorations impinging on the gingival margin. Those with subgingival margins were prone to more clinical attachment loss and this occurred in the first few years of restoration placement (Schätzle et al. 2001). Where overhangs of restorations were present, inflammation and bleeding on probing has been found (Lang et al. 1983), with more gingival inflammation and bone loss found near restorations (Albandar et al. 1995). Some studies have shown the presence of higher bacterial counts near composite restorations (Paolantonio et al. 2004), whilst others found non-precious metals and acrylic restorations associated with periodontal breakdown (Ababnaeh et al. 2011). Crowns with subgingival margins have been associated with an increase in periodontal pocket depth and attachment loss when compared to supragingival crown margins (Valderhaug and Birkeland 1976; Müller 1986; Reitemeier et al. 2002). Interproximal attachment loss has been found to be associated with caries and restorations; however, flossing showed a protective influence (Broadbent et al. 2006). Following the management of endodontic disease will be restoration of the tooth, and therefore, its impact on the periodontal tissues should not be forgotten.

The perio-endo interface is more complex. Periodontal disease and endodontic disease have been identified, studied and treated for centuries (Carranza et al. 2006; Hargreaves et al. 2011). Both have a variety of non-surgical and surgical care pathways, with the common goal of reducing the microbial load, in order to manage disease, and therefore, prevent eventual loss of the tooth.

The relationship between periodontal and pulpal disease was first described in 1964 (Simring and Goldberg 1964), when the effect of pulpal disease in the causation of, contribution to, and prevention of healing of periodontal disease was first demonstrated using a series of cases. At the time, this was termed 'retrograde' periodontitis (disease spreading from the apex of a root to the gingival margin) in order to differentiate it from marginal periodontitis (disease spreading from the gingival margin towards the apex of a root). It was thought that both micro-organisms and their toxins pass from the pulpal tissues to the periodontal tissues, with communications existing via neural pathways, lateral canals, dentinal tubules, the periodontal membrane, alveolar bone, apical foramen, vasculolymphatic drainage and dentinal permeability. It was also noted that both diseases have similar symptoms and signs, making diagnosis difficult. Simring and Goldberg (1964) reported a success rate of 89% for the 109 cases treated over 9 years using a variety of periodontal and endodontic treatment modalities. Although, much of the scientific understanding and rationale have not significantly changed, the methods of treatment and the order of treatment have marginally altered over the years, with emergence of some differing philosophies.

For both periodontal and endodontic disease, many classifications exist (Armitage 1999; Abbott and Yu 2007; European Federation of Periodontology 2019). For the purposes of this book, the discussion will be limited to a broad definition of periodontal disease and endodontic disease. The basic principles can be extrapolated to other more intricate diagnoses. Periodontal disease or periodontitis, in this book, will be taken to mean the pathological breakdown of the periodontium (inflammation of the gingival tissues, leading to attachment loss and resorption of the alveolar bone as measured from the cemento-enamel junction of a tooth), as a result of infection (plaque and residing bacteria) and inflammation (host response to the presence of plaque and associated bacteria). Endodontic disease, in this book, will be used to describe the loss of vitality of a tooth leading to inflammation and infection within the root canal system, and periradicular tissues as a response to the infection and inflammation within the root canal system of a tooth (requiring non-surgical endodontic treatment), and will include teeth that have already been root canal treated and still continue to house infection either within the canal system or outside the canal system (requiring endodontic re-treatment or surgical endodontics).

The diagnosis and treatment of dental infections that have a combined periodontal and endodontic component is complex, with practitioners having limited confidence to save such teeth, considering them of 'poor' or 'hopeless' prognosis (Simring and Goldberg 1964; Herrera et al. 2018; Khandelwal et al. 2020). Despite this, there are advantages to maintaining natural teeth, even if periodontally and endodontically treated (Eliyas et al. 2018). When a tooth is lost, the alternative to accepting a space is providing one of a variety of prosthetic replacement options (Cohn 2005; Hargreaves et al. 2011; De Backer et al. 2007; Doyle et al. 2007; Torabinejad et al. 2007; John et al. 2007; Zitzmann et al. 2009). Accepting a space may still be a potential option as function has been said to be adequate with a shortened dental arch, as long as there are four opposing posterior units (Kayser 1981). Although a shortened dental arch was not shown to lead dysfunction or discomfort (Witter et al. 1990, 1994; Sarita et al. 2003a), an increased number of chewing strokes are needed for swallowing (Kayser 1981; Sarita et al. 2003b). The movement of adjacent teeth into the space has been shown to be clinically insignificant in periodontally healthy adult patients, with less than 20% of teeth moving more than 2 mm (Love and Adams 1971; Witter et al. 1987, 2001; Kiliaridis et al. 2000; Shugars et al. 2000; Craddock and Youngson 2004; Christou and Kiliaridis 2007). This may be different in periodontally susceptible patients. The options for replacing teeth are removable prostheses (dentures) and fixed prostheses (bridges or implant-retained crowns and bridges).

Removable prostheses are a largely reversible method of restoring spaces, however may not be ideal in patients with periodontal disease or recurrent carious lesions as poor oral hygiene and plaque trapping around the removable prosthesis may lead to the demise of the remaining dentition (Bergman et al. 1995; Do Amaral et al. 2010). There are a number of studies that assessed the association of removable partial dentures with periodontal breakdown, some finding that there was a deleterious effect (Bates and Addy 1978; Seemann 1963; Yusof and Isa 1994) and others finding that good oral hygiene and thoughtful design of connectors can ensure maintenance of healthy periodontal tissues (Bergman et al. 1982; Carlsson et al. 1965; Berg 1985; Petridis and Hempton 2001). There may be the added difficulty of impression making in the presence of greatly mobile and periodontally involved teeth. Patients may fail to internalise removable appliances and tend not wear these when only posterior teeth are missing (Jepson et al. 1995; Davenport et al. 2000; Knezović Zlatarić et al. 2003; Clark et al. 2004; Allen et al. 2008). No significant differences have been found in patient related outcomes with provision of a removable denture and acceptance of a shortened dental (Wolfart et al. 2005).

Bridges are well tolerated by patients; however, require the presence of suitable bridge abutments (Sonoyama et al. 2002; Szentpetery et al. 2005; Tan et al. 2005; Geiballa et al. 2016). Conventional bridgework will require tooth preparation, with a potential for de-cementation of restorations and need for recycling of restorations (Brägger et al. 2001). Approximately 30% of teeth may lose vitality at 10 years and 35% at 15 years after placement of various fixed-fixed conventional bridge designs (Cheung et al. 2005). Conventional fixed-fixed bridges have a 10-year probability of survival of 89% and 10-year probability of success of 71% (Tan et al. 2004). Cantilevered bridges have a reported survival of 82% and success rate of 63% at 10 years, with the most common cause of complications being loss of pulp vitality of the abutment tooth (Pjetursson et al. 2004). Adhesive bridgework requires little or no preparation, and the failure is simple de-cementation (Djemal et al. 1999; King et al. 2015), especially if cantilever designs are used. If fixed-fixed designs are used there is potential for caries development if one wing de-cements. The median survival for cantilever designs had been reported to be 9.8 years, and that for fixed-fixed designs 7.8 years (Djemal et al. 1999). 65% survival at 10 years had been reported when all designs of resin-retained bridges were pooled in a systematic review of retrospective and prospective cohort studies with a minimum follow-up time of 5 years (Pjetursson et al. 2008). More recently, 80% survival rates for resin-retained bridges at 10 years has been reported (King et al. 2015).

It is often considered 'ideal' to offer rehabilitation with implant-retained prostheses. These can work well, but may also be challenging, with difficulty achieving ideal aesthetics and potential risk of damage to other structures (Palmer 1999). The placement of dental implants requires sufficient bone volume and periodontal health. Long-term maintenance is essential (Goodacre et al. 1999, 2003; Brägger et al. 2001; De la Rosa et al. 2013; Atieh et al. 2013; Bidra et al. 2016; Tran et al. 2016). The reported survival rate at 10 years for implant-supported fixed partial dentures is 87%, that for implant-supported single crowns is 98% (Pjetursson et al. 2007). Emerging evidence suggests that 19–65% may develop peri-implant mucositis and 22% of implants may develop peri-implantitis (Derks and Tomasi 2015), the management of which is often difficult, and likely to be even more challenging in an aging population (Roccuzzo et al. 2021). Therefore, it is of advantage to maintain natural teeth, because in an elderly patient, who may develop dementia or Alzheimer's disease, whose oral health is maintained by carers, it is easier to extract a natural tooth than provide complex dentistry to treat peri-implant disease, when problems arise. Further thought may need to be given to conversion of complex fixed implant-retained prostheses into simpler removable implant-retained prosthesis during the early stages of diagnosis of deteriorating medical health, as the population ages. In patients with treated periodontal disease, the occurrence of peri-implantitis has been reported to be 16–25.5% (Ong et al. 2008). When endodontic treatment was compared with implant treatment, both showed similar rates of survival, however, with more interventions required for maintaining implant-retained prostheses than endodontically treated teeth (Iqbal and Kim 2007; Doyle et al. 2006; Hannahan and Eleazer 2008). Hence, saving a tooth of strategic importance may well be preferred and should always be considered, even if the alternative appears easier in the short-term (Zitzmann et al. 2010).

Accurate diagnosis facilitates treatment planning and determination of prognosis, which will aid the clinician and patient in making a decision as to whether complex periodontal and endodontic treatment would be of short, medium and long-term benefit. In order to understand perio-endo lesions, it is necessary to understand the development of both structures, their individual disease processes and as well as the available treatment options for the individual diseases. This book aims to describe periodontal and endodontic health and disease, and the potential for communication between the structures at the periodontic-endodontic interface. The various chapters of the book describes examination and special tests useful for diagnosis, and discusses treatment planning, treatment modalities, as well as the prognosis of such treatment for teeth with perio-endo lesions.

Learning Objectives:
1. Develop an understanding of the pulp and periodontal tissues in health.
2. Recognise the close relationship between periodontal and endodontic structures which may lead to perio-endo lesions.
3. Appreciate the limitations of special tests in diagnosis of perio-endo lesions.
4. Comprehend the treatment options for perio-endo lesions and their prognosis.
5. Be able to treatment plan for perio-endo lesions to achieve optimal outcomes.

References

Ababnaeh KT, Al-Omari M, Alawneh TN. The effect of dental restoration type and material on periodontal health. Oral Health Prev Dent. 2011;9(4):395–403.

Abbott PV, Yu C. A clinical classification of the status of the pulp and the root canal system. Aust Dent J. 2007;52(1 Suppl):S17–31.

Albandar JM, Buischi YA, Axelsson P. Caries lesions and dental restorations as predisposing factors in the progression of periodontal diseases in adolescents. A 3-year longitudinal study. J Periodontol. 1995;66:249–54.

Allen PF, Jepson NJ, Doughty J, Bond S. Attitudes and practice in the provision of removable partial dentures. Br Dent J. 2008;204:E2.

Armitage GC. Development of a classification system for periodontal diseases and conditions. Ann Periodontol. 1999;4:1–6.

Atieh MA, Alsabeeha NHM, Faggion CM Jr, Duncan WJ. The frequency of peri-implant diseases: a systematic review and meta-analysis. J Periodontol. 2013;84:1586–98.

Bates JF, Addy M. Partial dentures and plaque accumulation. J Dent. 1978;6(4):285–93.

Berg E. Periodontal problems associated with use of distal extension removable partial dentures--a matter of construction? J Oral Rehabil. 1985;12(5):369–79.

Bergman B, Hugoson A, Olsson CO. Caries, periodontal and prosthetic findings in patients with removable partial dentures: a ten-year longitudinal study. J Prosthet Dent. 1982;48(5):506–14.

Bergman B, Hugoson A, Olsson CO. A 25-year longitudinal study of patients treated with removable partial dentures. J Oral Rehabil. 1995;22(8):595–9.

Bidra AS, Daubert DM, Garcia LT, Gauthier MF, Kosinski TF, Nenn CA, Olsen JA, Platt JA, Wingrove SS, Chandler ND, Curtis DA. A systematic review of recall regimen and maintenance regimen of patients with dental restorations. Part 2: implant-borne restorations. J Prosthodont. 2016;25:S16–31.

Brägger U, Aeschlimann S, Bûrgin W, Hämmerle CHF, Lang NP. Biological and technical complications and failures with fixed partial dentures (FPD) on implants and teeth after four to five years of function. Clin Oral Implants Res. 2001;12:26–34.

Broadbent JM, Williams KB, Thomson WM, Williams SM. Dental restorations: a risk factor for periodontal attachment loss? J Clin Periodontol. 2006;33(11):803–10.

Carlsson GE, Hedegård B, Koivumaa KK. Studies in partial dental prosthesis. IV. Final results of a 4-year longitudinal investigation of dentogingivally supported partial dentures. Acta Odontol Scand. 1965;23(5):443–72.

Carranza F, Newman M, Takei H. Carranza's clinical periodontology. 10th ed. St. Louis: Elsevier Saunders; 2006.

Chen SY, Wang HL, Glickman GN. The influence of endodontic treatment upon periodontal wound healing. J Clin Periodontol. 1997;24:449.

Cheung GSP, Lai SCN, Ng RPY. Fate of vital pulps beneath a metal ceramic crown or bridge retainer. Int Endod J. 2005;38(8):521–30.

Christou P, Kiliaridis S. Three-dimensional changes in the position of unopposed molars in adults. Eur J Orthod. 2007;29:543–9.

Clark RKF, Radford DR, Fenlon MR. The future of teaching of complete denture construction to undergraduates in the UK: is a replacement denture technique the answer? Br Dent J. 2004;196(9):571–5.

Cohn SA. Treatment choices for negative outcomes with non-surgical root canal treatment: non-surgical retreatment vs. surgical retreatment vs. implants. Endod Top. 2005;11:4–24.

Craddock HL, Youngson CC. A study of the incidence of over eruption and occlusal interferences in unopposed teeth. Br Dent J. 2004;196:341–8.

Davenport JC, Basker RM, Heath JR, Ralph JP, Glantz P-O. Need and demand for treatment. Br Dent J. 2000;189(7):364–8.

De Backer H, Maele GV, Decock V, Van De Berghe L. Long-term survival of complete crowns, fixed dental prostheses, and cantilever fixed dental prostheses with posts and cores on root canal treated teeth. Int J Prosthodont. 2007;20:229–34.

De La Rosa M, Rodríguez A, Sierra K, Mendoza G, Chambrone L. Predictors of peri-implant bone loss during long-term maintenance of patients treated with 10mm implants and single crown restorations. Int J Oral Maxillofac Implants. 2013;28(3):798–802.

Derks J, Tomasi C. Peri-implant health and disease. A systematic review of current epidemiology. J Clin Periodontol. 2015;42(Suppl 16):S158–71.

Djemal S, Setchell D, King P, Wickens J. Long-term survival characteristics of 832 resin-retained bridges and splints provided in a post-graduate teaching hospital between 1978 and 1993. J Oral Rehabil. 1999;26:302–20.

Do Amaral BA, Barreto AO, Gomes Seabra E, Roncalli AG, Carreiro DFP, A, De Almeida EO. A clinical follow-up study of the periodontal conditions of RPD abutment and non-abutment teeth. J Oral Rehabil. 2010;37(7):545–52.

Doyle SL, Hodges JS, Pesun IJ, Law AS, Bowles WR. Retrospective cross sectional comparison of initial nonsurgical endodontic treatment and single-tooth implants. J Endod. 2006;32:822–7.

Doyle SL, Hodges JS, Pesun IJ, Baisden MK, Bowles WR. Factors affecting outcome of single tooth implants and endodontic restorations. J Endod. 2007;33(4):399–402.

Eliyas S, Briggs P, Gallagher JE. The options for a tooth that requires root canal treatment. Dent Update. 2018;45(3):182–95.

European Federation of Periodontology 2019. New classification of periodontal and peri-implant diseases. https://www.efp.org/fileadmin/uploads/efp/Documents/Campaigns/New_Classification/Guidance_Notes/report-02.pdf. Last accessed 21 July 2023.

Geiballa GH, Abubakr NH, Ibrahim YE. Patients' satisfaction and maintenance of fixed partial denture. Eur J Dent. 2016;10(2):250–3.

Goodacre CJ, Kan JY, Rungcharassaeng K. Clinical complications of osseointegrated implants. J Prosthet Dent. 1999;81(5):537–52.

Goodacre CJ, Bernal G, Rungcharassaeng K, Kan JY. Clinical complications with implants and implant prostheses. J Prosthet Dent. 2003;90(2):121–32.

Hannahan JP, Eleazer PD. Comparison of success of implants versus endodontically treated teeth. J Endod. 2008;34:1302–5.

Hargreaves KM, Cohen S, Berman LH. Cohen's pathways of the pulp. 10th ed. St. Louis: Mosby Elsevier; 2011.

Herrera D, Retamal-Valdes B, Alonso B, Feres M. Acute periodontal lesions (periodontal abscesses and necrotizing periodontal diseases) and endo-periodontal lesions. J Periodontol. 2018;89(Suppl 1):S85–S102.

Iqbal MK, Kim S. For teeth requiring endodontic treatment, what are the differences in outcomes of restored endodontically treated teeth compared to implant-supported restorations? Int J Oral Maxillofac Implants. 2007;22:96–116. Erratum in: Int J Oral Maxillofac Implants. 2008;23(1):56

Jepson NJ, Thomason JM, Steele JG. The influence of denture design on patient acceptance of partial dentures. Br Dent J. 1995;178(8):296–300.

John V, Chen S, Parashos P. Implant or the natural tooth – a contemporary treatment planning dilemma? Aust Dent J. 2007;52(1 Suppl):S138–50.

Kayser AF. Shortened dental arches and oral function. J Oral Rehabil. 1981;8:457–62.

Khandelwal A, Billore J, Gupta B, Jaroli S, Agrawal N. Knowledge, attitude and perception on endo-perio lesions in practicing dentists - a qualitative research study. J Adv Med Dent Sci Res. 2020;11(8):31–4.

Kiliaridis S, Lyka I, Friede H, Carlsson GE, Ahlqwist M. Vertical position, rotation, and tipping of molars without antagonists. Int J Prosthodont. 2000;13:480–6.

King PA, Foster LV, Yates RJ, Newcombe RG, Garrett MJ. Survival characteristics of 771 resin-retained bridges provided at a UK dental teaching hospital. Br Dent J. 2015;218:423–8.

Knezović Zlatarić D, Celebić A, Valentić-Peruzović M, Jerolimov V, Pandurić J. A survey of treatment outcomes with removable partial dentures. J Oral Rehabil. 2003;30(8):847–54.

Lang NP, Kiel RA, Anderhalden K. Clinical and microbiological effects of subgingival restorations with overhanging or clinically perfect margins. J Clin Periodontol. 1983;10(6):563–78.

Love WD, Adams RL. Tooth movement into edentulous areas. J Prosthet Dent. 1971;25:271–8.

Müller HP. The effect of artificial crown margins at the gingival margin on the periodontal conditions in a group of periodontally supervised patients treated with fixed bridges. J Clin Periodontol. 1986;13(2):97–102.

Ong CT, Ivanovski S, Needleman IG, Retzepi M, Moles DR, Tonetti MS, Donos N. Systematic review of implant outcomes in treated periodontitis subjects. J Clin Periodontol. 2008;35(5):438–62.

Palmer R. Introduction to dental implants. Br Dent J. 1999;187(3):127–32.

Paolantonio M, D'ercole S, Perinetti G, Tripodi D, Catamo G, Serra E, Bruè C, Piccolomini R. Clinical and microbiological effects of different restorative materials on the periodontal tissues adjacent to subgingival class V restorations. J Clin Periodontol. 2004;31(3):200–7.

Petridis H, Hempton TJ. Periodontal considerations in removable partial denture treatment: a review of the literature. Int J Prosthodont. 2001;14(2):164–72.

Pjetursson BE, Tan K, Lang NP, Brägger U, Egger M, Zwahlen M. A systematic review of the survival and complication rates of fixed partial dentures (FPDs) after an observation period of at least 5 years. IV. Cantilever or extension FPDs. Clin Oral Implant Res. 2004;15:667–76.

Pjetursson BE, Brägger U, Lang NP, Zwahlen M. Comparison of survival and complication rates of tooth-supported fixed dental prostheses (FDPs) and implant- supported FDPs and single crowns (SCs). Clin Oral Implants Res. 2007;18(S3):97–113.

Pjetursson BE, Tan WC, Tan K, Brägger U, Zwahlen M, Lang NP. A systematic review of the survival and complication rates of resin-bonded bridges after an observation period of at least 5 years. Clin Oral Implant Res. 2008;19:131–41.

Reitemeier B, Hänsel K, Walter MH, Kastner C, Toutenburg H. Effect of posterior crown margin placement on gingival health. J Prosthet Dent. 2002;87(2):167–72.

Roccuzzo A, Stähli A, Monje A, Sculean A, Salvi GE. Peri-implantitis: a clinical update on prevalence and surgical treatment outcomes. J Clin Med. 2021;10:1107.

Sarita PT, Kreulen CM, Witter D, Creugers NH. Signs and symptoms associated with TMD in adults with shortened dental arches. Int J Prosthodont. 2003a;16:265–70.

Sarita PT, Witter DJ, Kreulen CM, Van't Hof MA, Creugers NH. Chewing ability of subjects with shortened dental arches. Community Dent Oral Epidemiol. 2003b;31:328–34.

Schätzle M, Land NP, Anerud A, Boysen H, Bürgin W, Löe H. The influence of margins of restorations of the periodontal tissues over 26 years. J Clin Periodontol. 2001;28(1):57–64.

Seemann SK. A study of the relationship between periodontal disease and the wearing of partial dentures. Aust Dent J. 1963;8(3):206–8.

Shugars DA, Bader JD, Phillips SW Jr, White BA, Brantley CF. The consequences of not replacing a missing posterior tooth. J Am Dent Assoc. 2000;131:1317–23.

Simring M, Goldberg M. The pulpal pocket approach: retrograde periodontitis. J Periodontol. 1964;35:22–48.

Sonoyama W, Kuboki T, Okamoto S, Suzuki H, Arakawa H, Kanyama M, et al. Quality of life assessment in patients with implant-supported and resin-bonded fixed prosthesis for bounded edentulous spaces. Clin Oral Implants Res. 2002;13:359–64.

Szentpetery AG, John MT, Slade GD, Setz JM. Problems reported by patients before and after prosthodontic treatment. Int J Prosthodont. 2005;18:124–31.

Tan K, Pjetursson BE, Lang NP, Chan ESY. Systematic review of the survival and complication rates of fixed partial dentures (FDPs) after an observation period of at least 5 years. – III. Conventional FDPs. Clin Oral Implants Res. 2004;15:654–66.

Tan K, Li AZ, Chan ES. Patient satisfaction with fixed partial dentures: a 5-year retrospective study. Singap Dent J. 2005;27(1):23–9.

Torabinejad M, Anderson P, Bader J, Brown LJ, Chen LH, Goodacre CJ, Kattadiyil MT, Kutsenko D, Lozada J, Patel R, Petersen F, Puterman I, White SN. Outcomes of root canal treatment and restoration, implant-supported single crowns, fixed partial dentures, and extraction without replacement: A systematic review. J Prosthet Dent. 2007;98(4):285–311.

Tran DT, Gay IC, Diaz-Rodriguez J, Parthasarathy K, Weltman R, Friedman L. Survival of dental implants placed in grafted and nongrafted bone: a retrospective study in a university setting. Int J Oral Maxillofac Implants. 2016;31(2):310–7.

Valderhaug J, Birkeland JM. Periodontal conditions in patients 5 years following insertion of fixed prostheses. Pocket depth and loss of attachment. J Oral Rehabil. 1976;3(3):237–43.

Witter DJ, Van Elteren P, Kayser AF. Migration of teeth in shortened dental arches. J Oral Rehabil. 1987;14:321–9.

Witter DJ, Cramwinckel AB, van Rossum GM, Käyser AF. Shortened dental arches and masticatory ability. J Dent. 1990;18(4):185–9.

Witter DJ, De Haan AF, Kayser AF, Van Rossum GM. A 6-year follow-up study of oral function in shortened dental arches. Part II: craniomandibular dysfunction and oral comfort. J Oral Rehabil. 1994;21:353–66.

Witter DJ, Creugers NH, Kreulen CM, De Haan AF. Occlusal stability in shortened dental arches. J Dent Res. 2001;80:432–6.

Wolfart S, Heydecke G, Luthardt RG, Marre B, Freesmeyer WB, Stark H, et al. Effects of prosthetic treatment for shortened dental arches on oral health- related quality of life, self-reports of pain and jaw disability: results from the pilot-phase of a randomized multicentre trial. J Oral Rehabil. 2005;32:815–22.

Yusof Z, Isa Z. Periodontal status of teeth in contact with denture in removable partial denture wearers. J Oral Rehabil. 1994;21(1):77–86.

Zitzmann NU, Krastl G, Hecker H, Walter C, Weiger R. Endodontics or implants? A review of decisive criteria and guidelines for single tooth restorations and full arch reconstructions. Int Endod J. 2009;42(9):757–74.

Zitzmann NU, Krastl G, Hecker H, Walter C, Waltimo T, Weiger R. Strategic considerations in treatment planning: deciding when to treat, extract, or replace a questionable tooth. J Prosthet Dent. 2010;104:80–91.

The Periodontic-Endodontic Interface

Abstract

This chapter considers the interface between the periodontal and endodontic architecture. The periodontic-endodontic interface is an intricate and complicated biological structure, combining and periodontium and endodontium. There are intimate communications and sophisticated messaging between varieties of cells, all aiming to maintain the balance of health. The following short summary of the embryonic development of the tooth helps to demonstrate this close relationship.

Embryological Development of the Tooth

At about 37 days of embryonic development, horseshoe shaped bands of odontogenic epithelium (the primary epithelial band) forms what will be the future upper and lower jaws, and give rise to two subdivisions of ectomesenchyme. The first of which is the dental lamina, and then just in front, the vestibular lamina (Nanci 2008). Localised thickenings (placodes) within the primary epithelium band initiates tooth families. The down growing dental lamina forms a series of epithelial outgrowths and ectomesenchymal cells accumulate around these outgrowths. Tooth development is catergorised into bud, cap and bell stages, although there is no clear demarcation between each stage. Each stage involves proliferation of cells with complex gene expression and signaling. The epithelial outgrowth becomes the enamel organ (resembling a cap) and ultimately forms the enamel of the tooth. The ectomesenchymal cells are the dental papilla and will form the dentine and pulp. The dental follicle or sac is made up of the condensed ectomesenchymal cells, which encapsulate the enamel organ and separate it from the dental papilla, and eventually this becomes the supporting structures of the tooth (Nanci 2008).

During the bell stage, the dental lamina disintegrates and separates the developing tooth from the oral epithelium. When the tooth erupts into the oral cavity, the

S. Eliyas, *The Periodontic-Endodontic Interface*,
https://doi.org/10.1007/978-3-031-49937-1_2

integrity between the tooth and the oral epithelium is re-established by the formation of a seal, the junctional epithelium. The blood vessels entering the dental papilla are clustered into groups and coincide with the position of the future roots. The initial growth of nerves into the dental papilla does penetrate the pulp, and are thought to be concerned with sensory innervation of the periodontal ligament and pulp (Nanci 2008). Also during the bell stage, the shape of the tooth is determined by morphodifferentiation, and the undifferentiated ectomesenchymal cells histodifferentiate into ameloblasts and odontoblasts. The dentine forming odontoblasts form an organic matrix, while moving towards the centre of the dental papilla, leaving a cytoplasmic extension. The matrix eventually mineralises around this cytoplasmic extension, and these form the dentinal tubules within dentine. Ameloblasts produce an organic matrix (which immediately mineralises) against this newly formed dentine, and move away from the dentine creating an increasingly thick layer of enamel (Nanci 2008).

Following completion of the crown formation, the epithelial cells of the inner and outer enamel epithelium proliferate from the cervical loop of the enamel organ to form a double layer of cells (the Hertwig's epithelial root sheath), which surrounds the dental pulp and carries on surrounding the pulp as the pulp expands. Ectomesenchymal cells at the periphery of the pulp, that faces the Hertwig's root sheath, differentiate into odontoblasts and form root dentine. Hertwig's root sheet extends around each apical foramen of a multirooted tooth, and anomalies in splitting of the primary apical foramen (which will become the pulp chamber) into secondary apical foramen (which will become the separate roots) give rise to pulpo-periodontal communications such as large furcal canals. This splitting of Hertwig's root sheath within roots to give rise to additional or accessory canals may not necessarily be an abnormality, as most teeth are now known to have complex root canal anatomy rather than one or two large canals (Ahmed and Hashem 2016). Hertwig's root sheath disintegrates as the root forms, but may leave clusters of cells behind, surrounded by a basal lamina, named the cell rests of Mallasez. These remain in the periodontal ligament and were originally thought only to give rise to cysts, however, are now thought to also take part in periodontal repair and regeneration (Nanci 2008).

The dental follicle is a fibrocellular layer surrounding the enamel organ and the dental papilla. It is thought that cementoblasts develop from differentiation of ectomesenchymal cells of the dental follicle and from some of the cells of the disintegrating Hertwig's root sheath. Cementoblasts form an organic matrix into which the collagen fibres of the periodontal ligament become anchored. Periodontal ligament cells, collagen fiber bundles, and the bone into which these fibres are embedded, are thought also to differentiate from the dental follicle (Nanci 2008).

The Perio-Endo Interface in Health

The perio-endo interface in health consists of the connections from the alveolar bone to the tooth via Sharpey's fibres and collagen fibres, fibroblasts and cementoblasts, acellular cementum, cellular cementum with cementocytes, Tomes granular layer (hypomineralised area of radicular dentine), dentine, predentine, and odontoblasts, which surrounds the neurovascular bundle of the pulp tissue. An intimate continuum is present between pulp-dentine complex and periodontal tissues with potential for communication via the apical foramen, dentinal tubules, lateral root canals, furcation root canals and fracture lines within the root structure (Fig. 2.1).

Tissues of the Periodontium

The supporting tissues of the periodontium include soft tissues (the marginal gingivae, the attached gingivae, the sulcular and junctional epitherlium, and periodontal ligament and connecting fibres) and hard tissues (cementum and bone).

The Periodontal Soft Tissues

Gingivae

The marginal gingivae is unattached and demarcated from the attached gingivae, usually by the free gingival groove. The 'V' shaped crevice between the unattached marginal gingivae and the tooth is the gingival sulcus, and can be probed with a

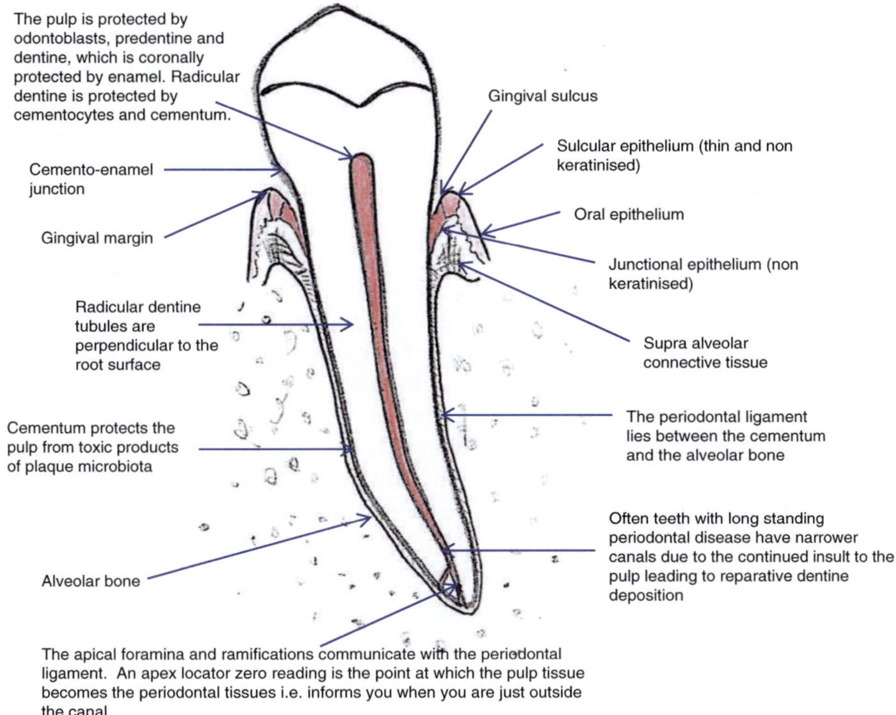

Fig. 2.1 The perio-endo interface

periodontal probe. The gingival sulcus (from the free surface of the junctional epithelium coronally to the level of the free gingival margin) varies from 0.5 to 4 mm (biological width), with any depth greater being considered pathologic. The depth of the gingival sulcus in health is variable from person to person, tooth to tooth, and tooth site to tooth site (Carranza et al. 2006; Schmidt et al. 2013). Deeper periodontal pockets should be treated with suspicion, and causes identified for optimal treatment and outcomes. This biological width is protective against periodontal breakdown, and if this width is encroached upon, it will re-establish more apically, leading to recession (Schmidt et al. 2013).

The attached gingiva is tightly bound to the underlying periodontium and alveolar bone, and extends to the more mobile oral mucosa (demarcated by the mucogingival junction). The mucogingival junction remains stationary throughout life, therefore, any reduction in the width of the alveolar mucosa occurs as a result of changes at the coronal aspect. The width of the attached gingivae, which is variable from person to person and varies in different parts of the same mouth, is not the same as the width of the keratinised tissue, as the keratinised mucosa also includes the unattached marginal gingivae.

Epithelium

The sulcular epithelium is a semi-permeable membrane and allows tissue fluid to seep into the sulcus and also bacterial products to permeate into the gingivae. The junctional epithelium is self-renewing, provides an efficient barrier against periodontal pathogens and is attached to the tooth surface by hemidesmosomes, gingival fibres as well as organic strands from the enamel. The surface cells of the junctional epithelium attach the gingivae to the tooth. They can also attach to afibrillar cementum if it is present on the crown of the tooth. The junctional epithelium forms a collar around the tooth and is 15–30 cells thick at the floor of the gingival sulcus and tapers apically to be 3–4 cells thick (Nanci and Bosshardt 2006; Nanci 2008).

The Periodontal Ligament

The periodontal ligament fibres surrounds the root surface and connects it to the alveolar bone, communicating with the bone marrow spaces. The periodontal ligament is a connective tissue with cells (including osteoblasts and osteoclasts), an extracellular component together with ground substance. The periodontal ligament is highly vascularized, and ranges from a width of 0.15–0.38 mm, with the thinnest portion around the middle third of the root, and its width may decrease with age (Nanci and Bosshardt 2006; Nanci 2008). The periodontal ligament is continually remodeling and is able to repair and regenerate, with the cells of the periodontal ligament contributing to the formation and resorption of alveolar bone and cementum (Carranza et al. 2006; Nanci and Bosshardt 2006).

The Periodontal Hard Tissues

Cementum

Cementum can be classified according to the time of formation (primary or secondary), the presence of cells within the cementum (acellular or cellular), and the origin of the fibres within the cementum (intrinsic fibres from the cementum or extrinsic fibres from the periodontal ligament). Acellular cementum provides attachment for the tooth, and cellular cementum is adaptive in response to toothwear and movement (Nanci 2008). Cementum, even in health, is permeable; there is transport of mineral through the cementum (Wassermann et al. 1941; Petelin et al. 1999), with cytoplasmic processes of cementum sharing a common border with dentinal tubules (Carranza et al. 2006). Sharpey's fibres being uncalcified cores in cellular cementum can create fibrinous communications into the periphery of dentine (Furseth 1974; Dongari and Lambrianidis 1988). If these Sharpey's fibres breakdown, a surface with micro-channels will be left allowing microbes and toxins to enter the dentinal tubules. Cementum can be missing due to recession, developmental grooves, resorption, periodontal disease as well as periodontal treatment (Chapple and Lumley 1999).

Bone

The alveolar process is the bone of the mandible and maxilla. It is comprised of compact cortical bone and central trabecular bone, with a lining of alveolar bone in the sockets. This alveolar bone is called bundle bone because periodontal ligament fibres form attachment to it via Sharpey's fibres. The cortical bone is thinner in the maxilla and thicker on the buccal aspects of the mandible. Thin bone is likely to resorb faster than thick bone in the presence of inflammation and infection. Trabecular bone can be missing around the anterior teeth, and here, the alveolar bone and cortical bone will be fused together. Alveolar bone is always remodeling in response to masticatory forces, has a high rate of turnover and is lost when the tooth is extracted (Nanci and Bosshardt 2006).

Tissues of the Endodontium

The endodontium or pulp-dentine complex consists of the soft pulpal tissues containing the odontoblasts living in the inner (pulpal) surface of the dentine (extending their processes towards the enamel-dentinal junction or cemento-dentinal junction), and the hard dentinal tissue.

The Endodontic Hard Tissues

Dentine

Dentine is hard tissue, which is protected by enamel and is in close contact with the pulp. Dentine consists of 70% inorganic material (hydroxyapatite), 10% water and 20% organic matrix (mostly type I collagen and ground substance: proteoglycans and glycoproteins). Dentinal tubules occupy 20–30% of the volume of intact dentine. Although odontoblasts themselves do not get embedded in their products, they leave a long process in the dentinal tubules, which extend approximately one third as far as the amelodentinal or cementodentinal junctions, with the rest of the dentinal tubule being filled with extracellular fluid (Whyman 1988; Gutman 1978; Zehnder et al. 2002). Dentine has been classified into primary, secondary and tertiary dentine, with further division into intertubular, peritubular and interglobular dentine, as well as coronal and root dentine.

Primary dentine forms during tooth development before eruption, is ordered, lines the pulp chamber as circumpulpal dentine, and has an outer layer of mantle dentine near cementum or enamel. The mantle dentine is different from the rest of the dentine in the way it is mineralised and the relationships between the collagenous and non-collagenous matrix (Nanci 2008).

Secondary dentine forms physiologically after the root is fully developed as peritubular dentine (which forms on the inside of tubules, has fewer collagen fibres and has a higher proportion of mineral), as intertubular dentine (which makes up the bulk of dentine, with collagen fibres that are at right angles to tubules, giving tensile strength), or as interglobular dentine; which is an organic matrix which remains unmineralised (Nanci 2008; Hargreaves et al. 2011).

Tertiary dentine forms as a response to insult. This may be 'reactionary', i.e. slow insult leading to the production of dentine by odontoblasts, and is similar to secondary dentine with some irregularity in tubule direction. Or, it may be 'reparative' as a result of fast insult destroying the odontoblasts. These destroyed cells are then replaced by cells of the cell rich layer, which are able to differentiate into odontoblast like cells, producing a very irregular, less tubular and is less mineralised dentine; a layer which therefore, is more permeable (Hargreaves et al. 2011).

Sclerotic dentine develops with age and in response to stimuli, causing partial or complete obliteration of dentine tubules. This reduces the permeability of dentine, protecting the pulp. In ageing, the formation of peritubular dentine is accelerated, and in pathology, dentine tubules are blocked by precipitation of hydroxyapatite and Whitlock crystals within the tubules (Hargreaves et al. 2011).

Dentinal tubules are widest closer to the pulp, and narrowest near the cementum, where they are sealed with cementum (Zehnder et al. 2002). Root dentine tubules are straight and about 1–3 microns in diameter (becoming narrower with age and insult, as a result of periradicular dentine formation). The number of tubules may be as high as 8000 per mm^2 at the cemeto-enamel junction and 57,000 per mm^2 at the pulpal end. In the cervical area, there may be as much as 15,000 dentinal tubules per mm^2. It has been reported that, when the cervical cementum is damaged, dentinal tubule exposure can occur in 18% of molars and 25% of anterior teeth (Rotstein and Simon 2004). The total density of tubules is less in the apical third (Zehnder et al. 2002). Most lateral and accessory canals are in the apical third of the root, with 30–40% of teeth having them (Hargreaves et al. 2011). Furthermore, furcation accessory canals may also be present in 23–76% of teeth (Hargreaves et al. 2011). The root has fewer dentinal tubules. The presence of dentinal fluid flowing out of the dential tubules reduces the movement of plaque and periodontal bacteria into the pulp (Zehnder et al. 2002). It must be remembered that dentinal tubules are 1–4 microns in diameter, whereas, most microbes are less than 1 micron in diameter, therefore, even small injuries to the cementum can lead to some bacterial contamination of the dentinal tubules.

The Endodontic Soft Tissues

Pulp

The pulp is a soft tissue also of mesenchymal origin, and is protected by predentine, with specialised odontoblasts, which are in direct contact with the dentine matrix. Even in mature teeth, the pulp is rich in stem cells, rendering it able to form dentine throughout life (i.e. indefinite potential for regeneration and repair). A vital pulp is considered healthy, with a good blood supply able to sustain life of the pulp-dentine complex. The loss of the blood supply will lead to death of the pulp. A non-vital pulp is sterile and would not lead to periodontal tissue destruction. However, once the necrotic pulp becomes infected, it may lead to widening of the periodontal ligament, apically or laterally (Bergenholtz 1974).

The pulp is a living structure within a hard tissue casing, capable of inflammatory/immune response to infective agents, and may not necessarily lead to the necrosis of the pulp. All stimuli reaching the pulp (hot, cold, pressure) are translated as pain by the pulp. The responses of the pulp to insults are cumulative leading to fibrosis, narrowing of the canal system, and development of calcifications (Hargreaves et al. 2011). The pulp will respond by the formation of sclerotic and reactionary dentine to protect itself, therefore, the root canals in patients with periodontal disease may be very narrow and haphazardley calcified (Bender and Seltzer 1972; Lantelme et al. 1976). Pulp calcifications have also been seen to be more prevalent in teeth with associated periodontal disease (Bender and Seltzer 1972), making endodontic treatment more challenging in these cases. The degree of inflammatory change and resultant narrowing of the canals with or without the development of pulp calcifications is dependent on the degree and duration of the periodontal disease, with 57% of teeth with periodontal disease showing alterations within the pulp (Bergenholtz and Lindhe 1978).

Like all other tissue in the body, the pulp reacts to irritation with inflammation (acute followed by chronic), and although inflammation itself is not a disease, it can be a manifestation of disease. It is an useful response, as it is the attempt by the body to fight against invading microbes. The causes of pulpal inflammation include microbial infection, any trauma that exposes the dentine tubules or cuts off the blood supply to the pulp (cutting dentine and vasoconstrictors can alter blood flow), prolonged extreme heat or cold, chemical agents (including bacterial toxins), pulpal tissue necrosis due to lack of oxygen or nutrients, and anachoresis (microbes entering from the bloodstream). The pulp has arterioles and venules (not arteries and veins), and there is fluid movement out of these during inflammation, which leads to an increase in pressure rather than volume. During inflammatory reactions of the pulp, this increase in tissue pressure leads to the death of odontoblasts, thereby, leading to migration of cells from the cell rich layer to the odontoblast layer, where they undergo mitosis to form new odontoblasts. Inflammation and local oedema also cause collapse of local microvasculature, compression of the tissue, with inflammation itself leading to local tissue hypoxia and tissue necrosis (the related pain is frequently described as throbbing). Relief of the pressure often alleviates the majority of the pain and extirpation of the inflamed pulp resolves the symptoms. If the cause of the inflammation is removed and the dentinal tubules are sealed, the pulp has the ability to form reparative dentine and recover.

Periodontal disease does not usually present with pain, therefore, if the patient presents with pain, endodontic involvement must be considered (Bender and Seltzer 1972). As well as increased intrapulpal pressure causing pulp death, it is also possible that this pressure pushes toxic products into the periodontal tissue through patent dentinal tubules, accessory canals and the apical foramen. This may cause some localised loss of attachment, which is reversible with endodontic treatment. If left untreated, however, it can become an established periodontal lesion (Anand et al. 2012).

The periodontal tissues and pulpal tissues have a common mesodermal origin. The dental papilla is the precursor for the dental pulp and dentine (the pulp-dentine complex), and the dental sac is the precursor for the supporting periodontal ligament. When Hertwig's epithelial root sheath separates the dental papilla from the dental follicle, at the late bell stage, it does not separate it entirely, maintaining a communication via the apical foramen (Nanci 2008). The pulp is enclosed entirely by dentine except at the apical foramina, which limits the pulp's ability to increase in volume during times of vasodilatation, hence blood flow must be carefully regulated. The blood flow to the pulp is through the main apical foramen as well as from some of the apical lateral canals and ramifications. The apical foramen reduces in diameter after tooth development is complete, can range from a diameter of 0.3–0.6 microns and is usually between 0.5 and 0.75 mm from the apex (Nanci 2008). The apical foramen is not a definite, single structure (Fig. 2.2), but has an apical constriction (considered the minor foramen) and beyond that the major

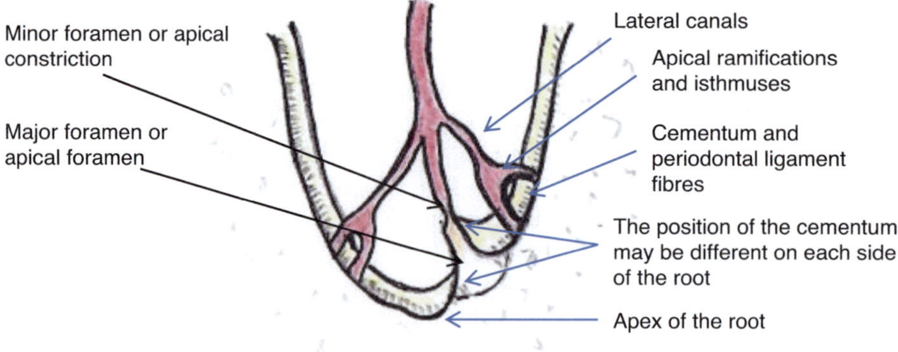

Fig. 2.2 The apical third of the root

foramen, which may be multiple and range from 0.2 – 3.8 mm from the apices of roots (Ricucci and Langeland 1998). The anatomy of the apex changes with age as cementum deposition increases. In older teeth and posterior teeth this distance can be larger. The major foramen maybe 0.3–0.5 mm away from the minor foramen (Gordon and Chandler 2004). It is not known how these distances may change with resorption and apical pathology.

Insults such as caries, trauma, large restorations, chemical and thermal stimulation, and periodontal disease may lead to pulpal inflammation and necrosis. As one would expect, numerous insults in the same tooth will lead to more inflammation and potential death of the pulp than one insult, and teeth with associated periodontal disease as well as caries, restorations or trauma, may have a higher degree of inflammation (Bender and Seltzer 1972). There has been some suggestion that mobility of teeth may also lead to pressure exerted on the blood supply through the apical foramen, leading to a reduced blood supply to teeth that are mobile (Bender and Seltzer 1972), potentially reducing the inflammatory response and permitting bacterial colonisation of the pulpal space. Periodontal disease leading to necrosis of the pulp, however, is rare (Bergenholtz and Lindhe 1978), and some studies have stated that the pulpal status may remain entirely independent of the periodontal status of a tooth (Czarnecki and Schilder 1979).

During root canal treatment, instrumentation and then obturation to the apical construction has been shown give the ideal outcomes (Ricucci and Langeland 1998). Therefore, the aim is always to complete root canal obturations to the apical constriction, however, this can be difficult as this area of the root may have a traditional/tapering/parallel constriction or have multiple constrictions (Fig. 2.3) or have an apex that is altogether disturbed by previous treatment or resorption (Dummer et al. 1984). It is not possible to consider the position of the cementum as the end point of the root canal as this can change with age and may be at different levels on different aspects of the same root (Ricucci 1998).

Ageing and the Tooth

In the young, the dentinal tubules are wider and the pulp is closer to the surface. Consequently, the effect of damage to the enamel (caries/erosion/operative procedures/trauma) and exposing dentinal tubules will have a greater effect on the pulp of a young person than that in an older person. With age, the pulp becomes less

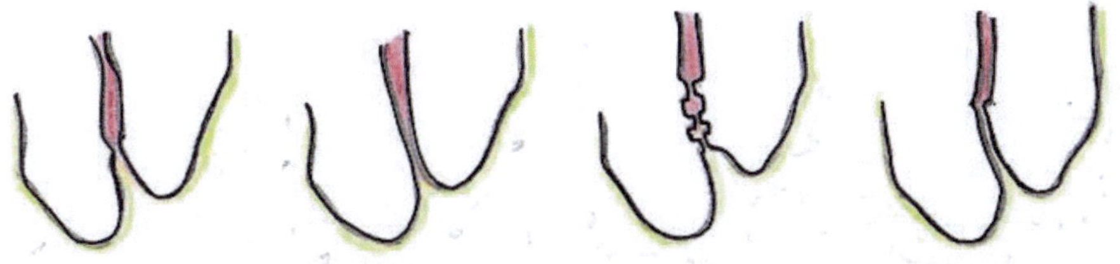

Fig. 2.3 Types of apical constriction as described by Dummer (Dummer et al. 1984)

cellular (due to cell deaths), more fibrous (as the surviving fibroblasts for a more fibrous matrix), there is less ground substance produced and it contains less water. Dentine deposition leads to reduction in the size of the pulp and there is a reduction in the fatigue life of a tooth, i.e. the tooth becomes more brittle (Hargreaves et al. 2011).

With age, the accessory canals also decrease in number (Thomas 1986), the apical foramina decrease in diameter, and due to the increased deposition of cementum, deviates from the long axis of the root (Kuttler 1955; Stein and Corcoran 1990). The laying down of sclerotic dentine leads to radicular dentine becoming less permeable (Nanci 2008; Carrigan et al. 1984; Kakoli et al. 2009), with some evidence that cementum may also become less permeable with age (Bennett and Miles 1955). In some ways this reduces the likelihood of pulpal pathology, however, this also makes endodontic treatment more challenging in the older tooth, especially if the teeth are not only heavily restored, but also periodontally involved.

Communication Between the Periodontium and Endodontium

Interaction between the periodontal architecture and the canal system of a tooth is necessary for connective tissue communications as well as vascular, lymphatic and neural communications (Table 2.1). In health, anatomical communication occurs via dentinal tubules, accessory canals, lateral canals and apical foramina (Abbott and Salgado 2009; Ricucci and Siqueira Jr. 2010; Chapple and Lumley 1999; Zehnder et al. 2002). In disease, endotoxins from within the root canal system can be transported to periaradicular tissues; inflammation can spread to periradicular tissues and cause bone resorption, and in very rare cases, microbes can spread into the bone itself, especially where the bone's ability to heal is impaired or there is immuno-compromise.

Table 2.1 Causes of communication between the periodontal and pulpal tissues

Developmental	Non-Developmental
Apical foramen – shared a common blood supply and vasculo-lymphatic drainage pathways as periodontal tissues	Root caries
	Cementum resorption due to periodontal disease and trauma
Lateral canals – may be present apically (30-40%) and furcally (23-76%) (Chapple and Lumley 1999)	Root fractures / cracks
Developmental grooves and extended radicular grooves	Cemental / cementodentinal tears
Hypoplasia or congenital absence of the cementum, thereby exposing the dentinal tubules	Iatrogenic perforations as a result of over instrumentation, root resorption, post preparation
Invaginations of the cementum-lined root	
Fissures and hypocalcifications of the cementum	Removal of the cementum with periodontal treatment
Dentine dysplasia type 1	Root resorption
Plaque traps like enamel pearls	

When dentine tubules are exposed, there is a communication between the oral cavity/periodontal tissues and the pulp. Other methods of communication between the periodontal and pulpal tissues are root caries/perforations/fractures, cementum resorption due to infections, radicular grooves/invaginatus, fissures and hypocalcifications within the cementum and dentine (Hargreaves et al. 2011). Furcal canals, like lateral canals and exposed dentinal tubules can lead to communication between the periodontal tissues and pulpal tissues, and interradicular inflammation of the periodontal tissues is possible when there is pulpal inflammation (Seltzer et al. 1963a, 1963b; Seltzer et al. 1967).

Exposure of Dentinal Tubules

Cementum is closely related to the dentine, and the border between the two is not distinct. Some studies have shown this border to have the presence of cementum, a cementodentinal junction (barrier) and dentine, with the cementodentinal junction found to be thinner in periodontally diseased teeth (Petelin et al. 1999). Normally, the tooth maintains an intact layer of cementum on the root surface. Dentinal tubules may be exposed if the cementum and enamel do not meet at the cementoenamel junction, or if the cementum or enamel is removed due to trauma, bleaching, scaling and root planing or root caries.

The pulp is not directly affected until the cementum is damaged and dentinal tubules are exposed to the oral cavity and pathogens, and still the pulp may not lose vitality unless the main blood supply to the pulp is affected, although, regression of the pulp in the areas of dentinal tubule exposure may be seen (Langeland et al. 1974). Theoretically, if there is damage to the cementum, and the dentinal tubules of the roots are exposed to healthy periodontal tissues, there is no influx of microbes. Where there is active periodontal disease, there is potential for microbes and toxins to reside within the periodontal tissues, and therefore, enter exposed dentinal tubules, thereby eventually entering the pulp tissue (Rubach and Mitchell 1964; Lindhe et al. 2008; Adriaens et al. 1988). Toxins from the periradicular tissues and exposed dentine may not reach the pulp easily due to dentinal fluid and the host response. Periodontal microbes only causes pulpal damage when major lateral canals become contaminated with plaque or when there is resorption and loss of the protective layer of cementum (Bergenholtz and Lindhe 1978).

Removal of cementum can allow bacteria to invade dentinal tubules, with more bacterial invasion occurring coronally than in the mid root and apex. Sclerosis of the dentinal tubules will inhibit invasion, as would the presence of salivary mucin and immunoglobulins. Some have supposed that 'proper root planing' would remove bacteria as well as a layer of cementum (Riffle 1953). Modern methods of scaling and root debridement can still remove cementum if not carefully administered, exposing dentine tubules and cause dentine hypersensitivity, which may last several weeks, and application of fluoride helps (Tammaro et al. 2000).

Lateral Canals, Apical Ramifications and the Apical Foramen

Lateral canals and apical ramifications are mainly found in the apical third of the root (74%), with less in the middle third (15%) and even less in the coronal third of roots (11%). These do not give a collateral blood supply to the tooth, except maybe in the apical 1–2 mm of the root (Ricucci and Siqueira Jr. 2010).

Apical ramifications and lateral canals usually house connective tissue and connect the blood supply of the pulpal tissues to the periodontal tissues, and have a significant resistance to bacteria. Although bacterial products may cause inflammation within the lateral canals and apical ramifications, there is only necrosis in the lateral canals if there is long-standing pulp necrosis in the main canal. If there is vital tissue in the main canal, there is vital tissue in the lateral canals, if there is inflamed tissue in the main canal, the tissue in the lateral canals and apical ramifications may also be inflamed, if there is necrotic pulp near the lateral canal or apical ramifications, there is only likely to be partial necrosis with possible bacteria within the lateral canals and apical ramifications. Depending on the chronicity of the necrotic pulp, the lateral canals may become infected with microbes. As the tissues in the lateral canal and apical ramifications are nourished by the rich blood supply from the periodontal tissues, any bacteria present are also nourished by the same blood supply. These canals and ramifications exit in to the periodontal ligament, however, the periodontal ligament will remain free of inflammation where there is good periodontal health. Although, it is possible for low molecular weight soluble products to diffuse through ramifications and lateral canals to induce or sustain inflammatory reactions in the periodontal tissues, and lead to bone resorption (Ricucci and Siqueira Jr. 2010).

The presence of a widened periodontal ligament or radiolucency in areas of the root other than the apex, should give suspicion to the presence of a lateral canal. In periodontally involved teeth, inflammation within the pulp has been related to the presence and number of lateral canals present (Bender and Seltzer 1972). Lateral periodontal lesions associated with ramifications are rare compared to how frequently teeth have these ramifications. This may be because the largest of these ramifications are still 3 times smaller than the mean diameter of the main apical foramen. Albeit relatively rare, toxins and inflammatory agents can lead to the presence of lateral periodontal lesions. These still heal once the bacteria within the main canal are removed, often because in early lesions, there may be no bacteria within the lateral canal itself (Bender and Seltzer 1972; Ricucci and Siqueira Jr. 2010). It is not possible to reach, clean, disinfect and fill most of these ramifications, unless sufficiently large, therefore, it is possible that unfilled lateral canals may be associated with post-treatment disease. Attempts should be made to fill ramifications that are large enough to harbor microbes, especially where these ramifications give microbes obvious access to the periradicular tissues. However, most teeth with ramifications too small to fill, still heal after root canal treatment despite not all of the ramifications being filled (Ricucci and Siqueira Jr. 2010).

In periodontal disease, when the subgingival flora reaches the lateral canals, the microcirculation is severed, yet the inflammation of the adjacent pulp can be minimal. In long standing lesions, bacteria and their products can enter lateral canals to cause pulpitis (Bender and Seltzer 1972), and, pulp necrosis only occurs after the blood supply to the main apical foramen has been compromised (Ricucci and Siqueira Jr. 2010). A relationship between the depth of periodontal pocket, degree of bone loss or extent of periodontal disease and the extent of pulpal inflammation has not been found. It has been suggested that molar teeth may have more perio-endo lesions due to the number of lateral and accessory canals present when compared to anterior teeth (Bender and Seltzer 1972).

When the subgingival biofilm reaches the apical foramen, there is irreversible damage to the blood supply, and therefore, the whole pulp becomes necrotic. In multi-rooted teeth, if only one root is involved, the other roots may continue to have a blood supply and the pulp chamber may still have vital tissue (Langeland et al. 1974; Ricucci and Siqueira Jr. 2010). The effects of ongoing periodontal treatment and other restorative dental treatment are cumulative, and therefore, in time teeth may lose vitality and require root canal treatment, even when the periodontal disease process has not breached the apical foramen (Anand et al. 2012).

Developmental Grooves and Disorders of the Cementum/Dentine

Grooves in the roots (radicular grooves) may develop during germination and as a result of fusion of developing teeth (Tagger 1975; Hülsmann et al. 1997; Aryanpour et al. 2002). Palatal/buccal grooves may extend anywhere from the cingulum to the apex of a root and can be classified into various forms (Kim et al. 2017). A reasonable classification to use is Type I: extending to the coronal third of the root, Type II: extending beyond the coronal third but is shallow and not involving the pulp tissue, and Type III: long and deep groove extending beyond the coronal third of the root and involving the pulpal tissue (Gu 2011). These are a developmental abnormality thought to be due to folding of the enamel organ and Hertwig's epithelial root sheath, as a result of attempts to develop another root, alteration of the genetic mechanism or a form of dens invaginatus (Kim et al. 2017). Like dens invaginatus, developmental grooves can harbor microbes, leading to the development of a periodontal pocket (Simon et al. 1971; Kim et al. 2017). If the periodontal lesion is long standing, or the groove extends to the pulp, it may lead to endodontic involvement and a perio-endo lesion. The palato-gingival groove has a prevalence of 1.9% to 8.5% and occurs in 4.4% of upper lateral incisors and 0.28% of upper central incisors (Hargreaves et al. 2011; Kim et al. 2017).

Any developmental disturbance in the mineralisation of cementum or dentine can lead to abnormal communication between the periodontium and the endodontium (Dongari and Lambrianidis 1988; Somerman et al. 1993; Seow 2014). For example, patients with Type 1 dentine dysplasia can have normally formed crowns of teeth, with no or rudimentary formation of the root due to a disturbance in dentine formation (Fulari and Tambake 2013; Ravanshad and Khayat 2006). This results in short/blunted roots, sclerosis of the pulp chamber and presence of periapical pathology. Early periodontal lesions can become perio-endo lesions as the apices of the roots are so close to the gingival margin. Enamel pears and bifurcation ridges can also act as plaque traps that may instigate periodontal breakdown in susceptible individuals (Dongari and Lambrianidis 1988).

X-linked hypophosphatemia is a metabolic disorder causing loss of phosphate through renal tubules, and thereby, reducing the circulating levels of calcium and phosphate (Case 1). The dentition is affected to varying degrees with a spectrum of afflictions including short roots, enlarged pulp chambers and prominent pulp horns, as well as thin bony trabeculae and loss of lamina dura as seen radiographically. Interglobular spaces are seen in the circumpulpal dentine as a result of a lack of fusion of calcospherites, and these spaces are filled with non-mineralised organic matrix. There can be hypoplastic enamel and large tubular clefts and lacunae extending along the dentino-enamel junction. Bacteria can enter and spread along these spaces and clefts leading to spontaneous apical abscesses, in the absence of caries or a history of trauma (Hanisch et al. 2019; Lee et al. 2017).

Case 1 A 42-year-old female patient presented in July 2018 with a history of periodontal disease on a background of x-linked hypophosphatemia. She had been previously treated for periodontal disease and endodontic disease. There was no history of trauma and the loss of her anterior teeth was related to endodontic infections. As can be seen from the Dental Panoramic Tomograph (DPT) the remaining dentition is minimally restored (with the exception of the canine teeth used as bridge abutments) and yet vertical bone loss has occurred (Fig. 2.4). The Long Cone Periapical (LCPA) radiographs show progression over time (Figs. 2.5a, b, 2.6a, b, 2.7a, b). The periodontal disease was disproportionate to the level of plaque present and the need for endodontic treatment is likely to be related to the easy spread of microbes within poorly mineralised dentine. Since 2018, although most areas improved, despite the patient's good oral hygiene following further periodontal treatment, the periodontal support around the upper molar and premolar teeth deteriorated rapidly and some of the molars were extracted (Figs. 2.8 and 2.9). Endodontic treatment did not appear to elongate the life of teeth, and this may be explained by bacterial contamination of the poorly mineralised dentine.

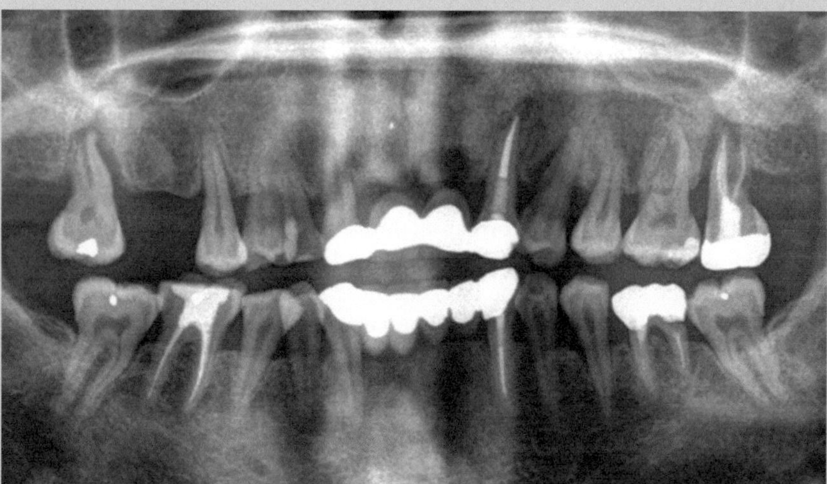

Fig. 2.4. DPT (2018) showing generalised horizontal bone loss, vertical bone defects and perio-endo lesions associated with the upper second molars, acquired loss of teeth, and anterior bridgework

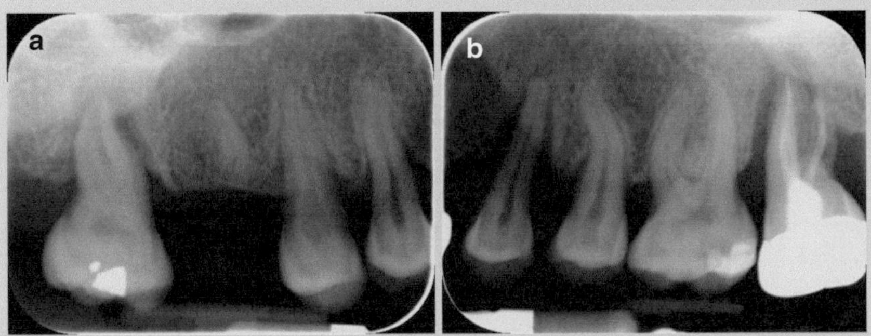

Fig. 2.5. LCPA radiographs of the right (**a**) and left (**b**) maxillary molars and premolars in July 2018

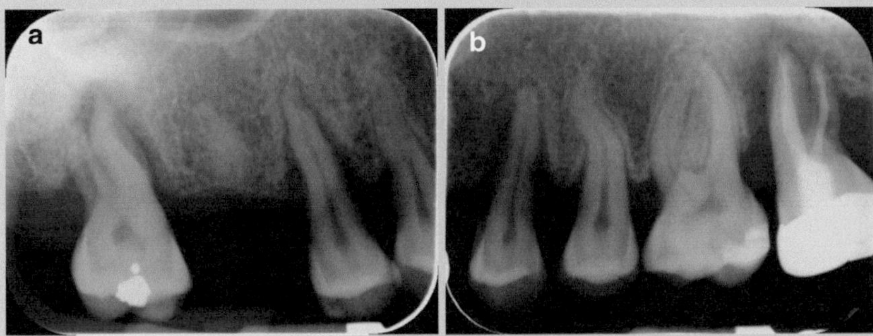

Fig. 2.6 LCPA radiographs of the right (**a**) and left (**b**) maxillary molars and premolars in October 2019

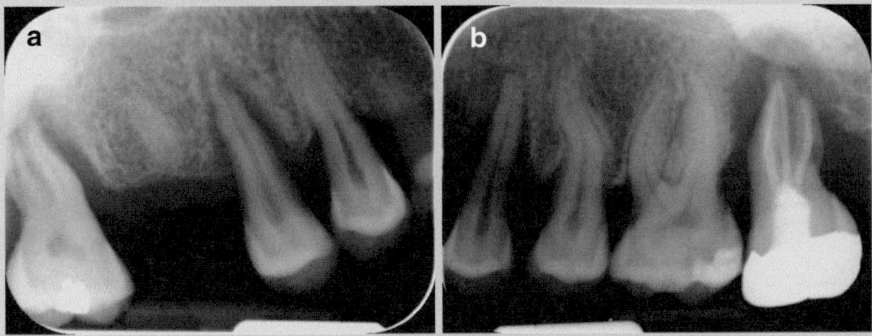

Fig. 2.7 LCPA radiographs of the right (**a**) and left (**b**) maxillary molars and premolars in January 2020

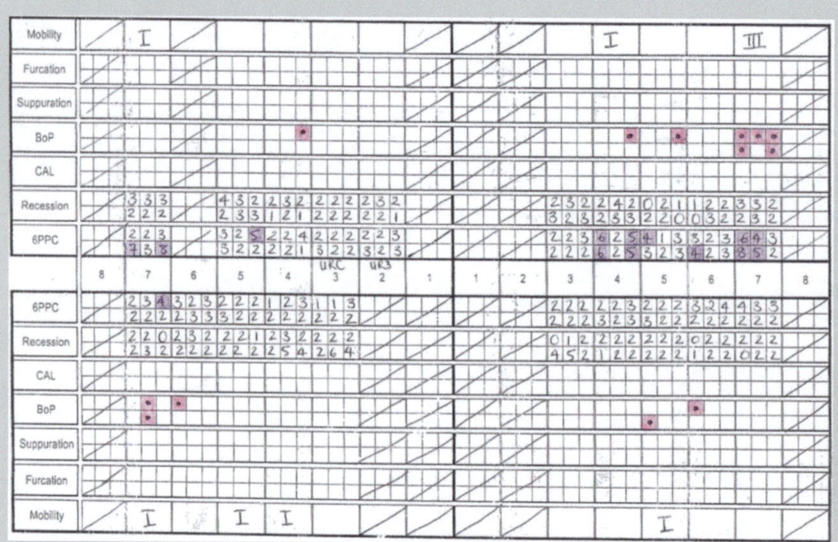

Fig. 2.8 Full periodontal indices taken in July 2018

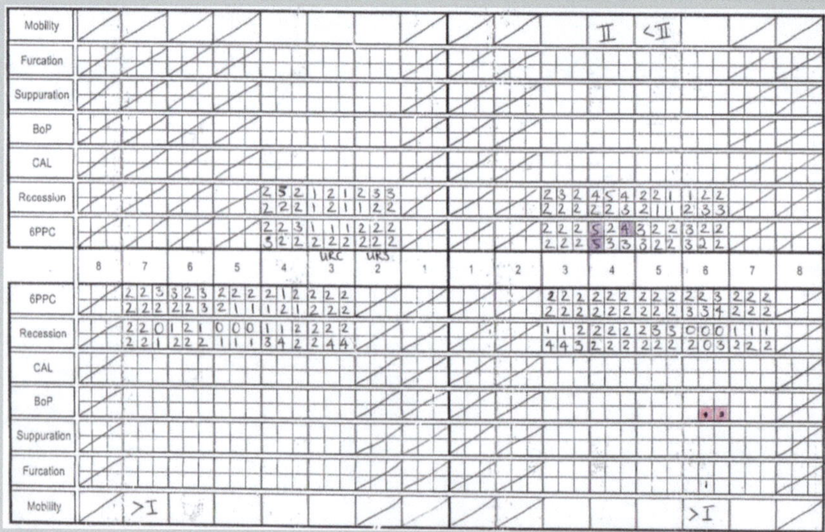

Fig. 2.9 Full periodontal indices taken in August 2020:

Perforations

Perforations are usually formed during endodontic treatment (47%), when instrumenting the canal, and post-endodontic treatment (53%) when preparing the canal for placement of a post (Farzaneh et al. 2004). Most have been found to be in maxillary teeth (73%) while 27% were found in the mandible. Often these are a result of the palatal inclination of teeth having been under estimated when preparing a canal to receive a post, due to overzealous instrumentation (strip perforations), or in the floor of the pulp chamber of multirooted teeth whilst trying to locate canals (Clauder and Shin 2009). Strip perforations may be more difficult to diagnose, and may only be considered when there is failure of healing following root canal treatment, unless obvious radiographically or due to bleeding intra-operatively. Perforation related to the placement of a post causes significant periodontal damage due to the size of a post in comparison to an endodontic file. Periodontal therapy may be required after post-related perforation repair.

Diagnosis of perforations may be possible clinically at the time of injury, and depending on the location, may be visible from within the canal with magnification (often seen as bleeding from within the canal, and once haemostasis is observed, the soft tissue may be visible) or radiographically (Case 2). Perforation of the root may cause instant pain even if the patient is under local anaesthesia, as the nerves of the periodontal ligament will be stimulated. Some perforations may require surgical repair, and healing of the periodontal tissues is likely to be through scar tissue formation.

This injury to the periodontal ligament can lead to inflammation, destruction of the periodontal ligament, bone resorption and proliferation of the epithelium, leading to a periodontal pocket. The length of time a perforation is left untreated will determine its outcome and chronic lesions are more likely to have developed epithelialised periodontal pockets, which are more difficult to resolve.

Case 2 A patient seen for root canal treatment of the UL2 had suffered a perforation during root canal treatment (Figs. 2.10 and 2.11). Although the apex locator zero reading was 11.5 mm, the working length radiograph had been taken with a file to 16.5 mm (Fig. 2.12a, b). Extension of the working length file beyond the perforation is likely to have damaged the periodontal ligament, however a periodontal pocket did not develop between appointments in this patient, as this patient appears not to be periodontally susceptible. The canal was found (Fig. 2.13a), the perforation was repaired (Fig. 2.13b) and the root canal was onturated (Fig. 2.13c). The apical area is healing without development of a periodontal pocket (Fig. 2.13d).

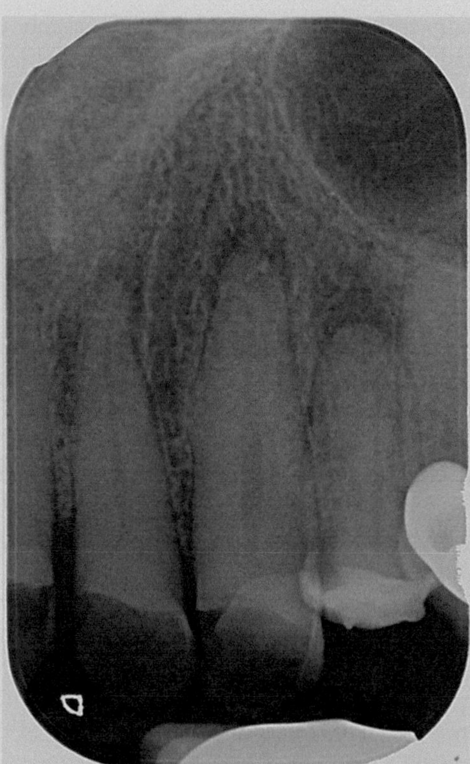

Fig. 2.10 Pre-operative LCPA radiograph of the UL234 with periapical pathology and a lateral radiolucency associated with the UL2. The canals in the UL2 and UL3 are visible on the radiograph

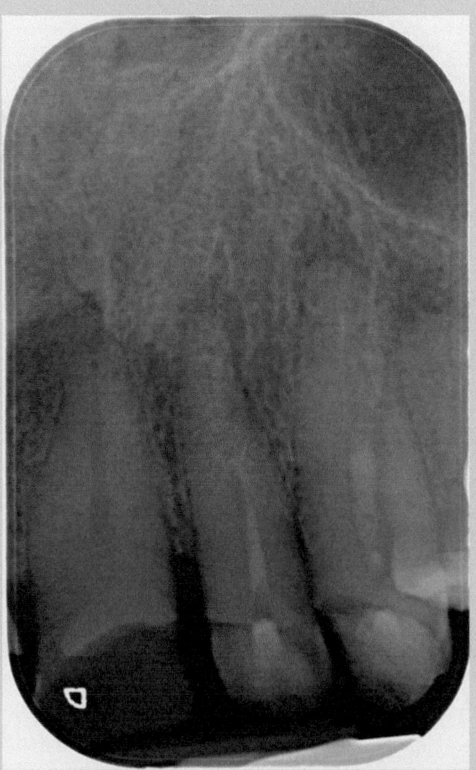

Fig. 2.11 LCPA radiographs following attempted root canal treatment of the UL23 with non-setting calcium hydroxide visible tracking to the lateral radiolucency associated with the UL2

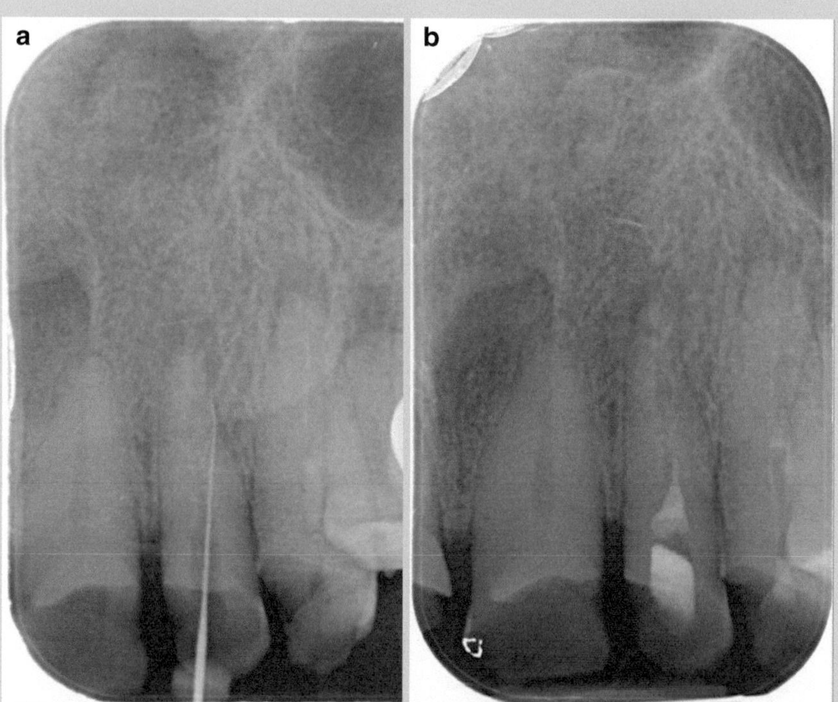

Fig. 2.12 LCPA (working length) radiograph of the UL2 with a #10 K-file in the perforation, tracking to the lateral radiolucency (**a**) and post temporisation with calcium hydroxide (**b**)

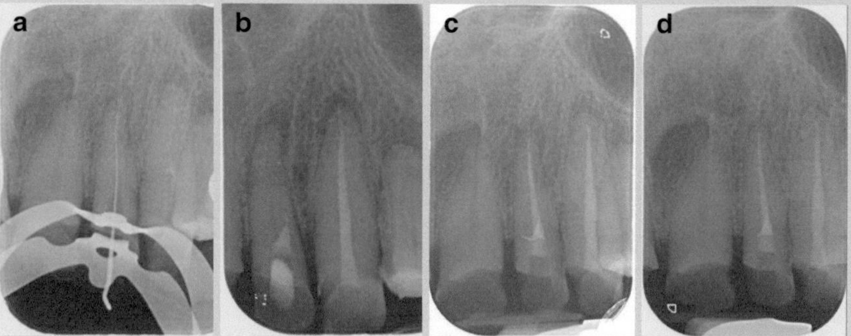

Fig. 2.13 LCPA radiographs of the UL2 with a #10 K-file in the canal (**a**), repair of the perforation with mineral trioxide aggregate or MTA (**b**), obturation of the canal (**c**) and review (**d**)

Root Fractures

Root fractures are present in vital and non-vital teeth, however may be more prevalent in root filled teeth (Zehnder et al. 2002). The fracture may have been the reason the tooth required endodontic treatment, or may be the result of restorative procedures, and reduced elasticity of dentine as a result of endodontic treatment. Although the loss of pulp or loss of moisture does not affect biomechanical properties of dentine, depletion of dentinal collagen may lead to less elastic dentine, which is more prone to shearing. Microbes and their products can also degrade collagen, as can Sodium hypochlorite in concentrations over 2%. There is a synergistic effect of Ethylenediaminetetraacetic acid (EDTA) and Sodium hypochlorite (NaOCl) when used together. Heat can dehydrate a tooth and denature collagen. Calcium hydroxide can reduce the flexural strength of dentine (Kishen 2006).

In anterior teeth, there is no difference in fracture susceptibility of root filled and non-root filled teeth (Trabert et al. 1978). In posterior teeth, endodontic procedures reduce tooth stiffness by 5%, the presence of an occlusal restoration can reduce the stiffness by 20% and the presence of a mesio-occlusal-distal restoration can reduce the stiffness by 63% (Reeh et al. 1989). In terms of providing endodontic treatment, the loss of marginal ridge and occlusal isthmus weakens teeth (Reeh et al. 1989; Mondelli et al. 1980), straight-line access may weaken adjacent cusps (Hansen and Asmussen 1993), post preparation removes radicular dentine (Trope and Ray 1992), excess force during canal obturation may propagate cracks (Pitts et al. 1983) and proprioception is thought to be reduced by 30% after endodontic treatment. Higher pain threshold are said to increase occlusal loads, however the presence of the periodontal ligament may provide some protection (Randow and Glantz 1986).

When a fracture is present within the crown of a tooth, it may lead to a piece of the enamel, or a piece of enamel and dentine being lost. When a fracture extends to the roof of the pulp chamber, the tooth may lose vitality and require endodontic treatment. When the fracture reaches the floor of the pulp chamber, it may be regarded as a vertical fracture of the tooth, rendering the tooth unrestorable. Root fractures may not only be detrimental and communicate with the marginal periodontal tissues, but when there is a vertical root fracture, they often appear as 'j-shaped' radiolucencies (Case 3) and render the tooth unrestorable. Horizontal root fractures often appears as a 'halo' on the radiograph (Case 4).

Case 3 In cases where there is minimal general horizontal bone loss, the development of a deep pocket should raise suspicion (Fig. 2.14). In this 65-year old male patient, who does only have 10–15% horizontal bone loss, the presence of a crack led to loss of vitality of the LL7, which eventually presented with a deep pocket and 'J-shaped' pattern of bone loss (Fig. 2.15). Looking at the first radiograph (Fig. 2.14), one may have confused this lesion to be of primarily periodontal origin, due to the periodontal susceptibility and the presence of calculus distally. When the patient then presented, a few weeks later, with a vertical fracture across from the mesial marginal ridge to the distal marginal ridge, in hindsight, the 'J-shaped' lesion (Fig. 2.15) was indicative of this fracture within the tooth.

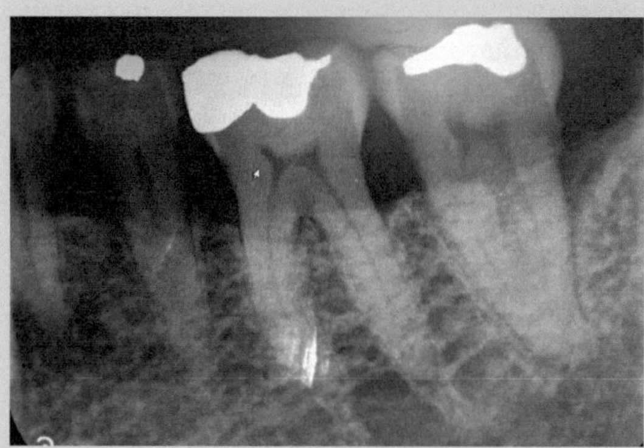

Fig. 2.14 LCPA radiograph of the LL567, revealing horizontal bone loss of 40% and early vertical bone defects associated with the distal aspect of the LL6 and a more marked vertical bone defect associated with the LL7. An artifact is present on the film at the level of the mesial root of the LL6

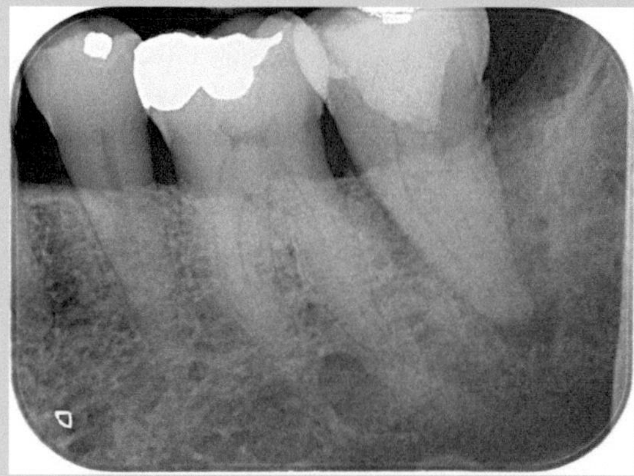

Fig. 2.15 LCPA of the LL567 revealed a radiolucency around the root of the LL7 which can be described as a 'j' shaped lesion

Case 4 A horizontal root fracture in the UL1 following a history of trauma. This female patient in her 30s presented with a draining sinus within the buccal attached gingivae of the UL1. The horizontal root fractured UL1 (Fig. 2.16a), without associated periodontal pocketing, resolved to some degree with endodontic treatment (Fig. 2.16b). In this case the canal was obturated with gutta percha. In such cases the draining sinus tends to resolve, however the periradicular radiolucency can remain, and may have healed with fibrous scar tissue Fig. 2.16c). This is likely to be a patient that is not periodontally susceptible.

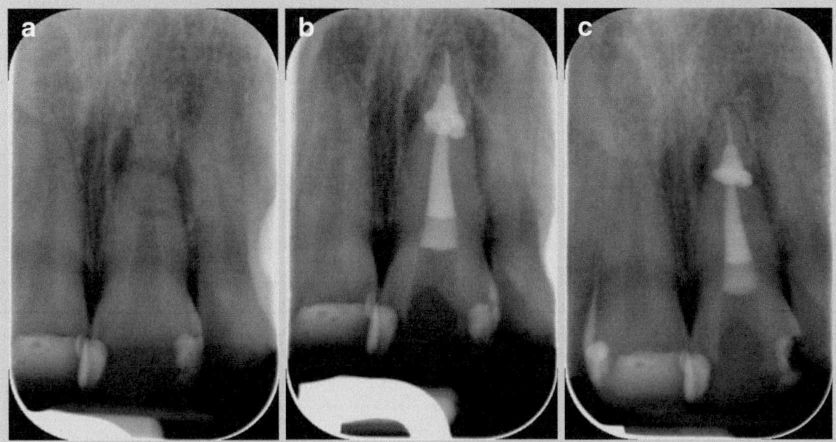

Fig. 2.16 LCAP radiograph of the UL1 (**a**) pre-operatively revealed a horizontal fracture in the root, (**b**) endodontic treatment was completed in June 2018 and (**c**) reviewed in June 2019

Cemental Tears

Cemental tears are considered a type of root fracture, where there is complete or partial detachment of the cementum from the dentino-cemental junction along the incremental line, and can cause periodontal defects/deep pockets potentially with endodontic involvement (Ong et al. 2019; Lin et al. 2011, 2012, 2014). The aetiology of cemental tears is unknown. Age, gender, tooth type, previous periodontal and endodontic treatment, trauma and excessive occlusal forces have been cited as potential causes. Cemental tears are more common in anterior teeth and more common on the mid and apical third of the root. Non-surgical periodontal/endodontic treatment of these lesions has been shown not to be as effective as surgical debridement, although recurrence is apparently possible (Keskin and Güler 2017; Jeng et al. 2018; Ong et al. 2019).

Tooth/Root Resorption

Resorption of roots may be internal or external, and is the physiological/pathological loss of tooth structure and sometimes bone, being replaced with bone, granulation tissue cementum or cementum like tissue (Lin et al. 2022; Abbott and Lin 2022). In order for resorption to occur, there must be a breach in the natural barriers in a tooth (for example periodontal and cementum cells along the external root, or odontoblasts in the predentine along the pulp), a stimulating factor that is continuous (bacteria, necrotic barrier cells, developmental defects, pathology like tumours), and a blood supply for the clastic cells (Abbott and Lin 2022). Internal resorption occurs when the odontoblastic layer and predentine are damaged (Rotstein and Simon 2004). If the continuous stimulating factor or the blood supply is the pulp, for example in internal resorption, the resorption usually resolves with endodontic treatment (Fig. 2.17a, b), and unless left untreated, is unlikely to involve the periodontal tissues.

External root resorption may be inflammatory (initiated by pulpal or sulcular infection), or non-inflammatory (invasive/cervical or replacement). Usually the presence of a layer of blast cells, such as cementoblasts, prevent and protect dental hard tissue from resorption, however, dental trauma, excessive orthodontic forces and aggressive scaling can damage this layer of cells, and initiate root resorption. In order for the resorptive process to continue, there needs to be a lasting osteoclast stimulus such as infection or continuous mechanical forces. External inflammatory root resorption may begin as a result of damage to the periodontal ligament cells, although, may continue as a result of a necrotic pulp; therefore, root canal treatment may still be indicated (Tronstad 1988). External inflammatory root resorption may be seen radiographically as loss of cementum, and/or loss of periodontal ligament space, with an adjacent radiolucency in the bone. Once the tooth is root canal treated, healing occurs, with the radiolucency filling in with bone (Fuss et al. 2003). Inflammatory external resorption resulting from infection is common, with almost all teeth with apical periodontitis exhibiting some degree of inflammatory resorption.

Replacement resorption leading to ankylosis (where the tooth is fused to the bone, without the presence of a periodontal ligament space) is the removal of the root structure (cementum, dentine and the periodontal ligament) by osteoclasts and deposition of bone tissue by osteoblasts (Tronstad 1988). Replacement resorption is usually induced by trauma resulting in death of cementum cells, and radiographically the lamina dura and periodontal ligament space is not visible (Fig. 2.18). Replacement resorption is difficult to halt, however, may be transient, and therefore, self-limiting. Some have said it may be possible to arrest and even reverse replacement resorption with regenerative

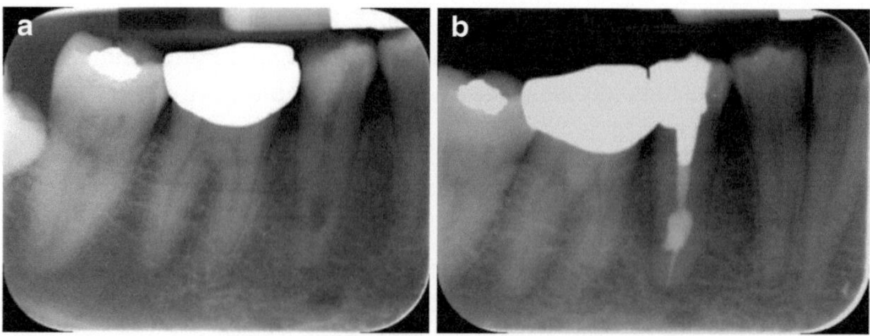

Fig. 2.17 LCPA radiograph of an internal resorptive defect in the LR5 before (**a**) and after (**b**) root canal treatment)

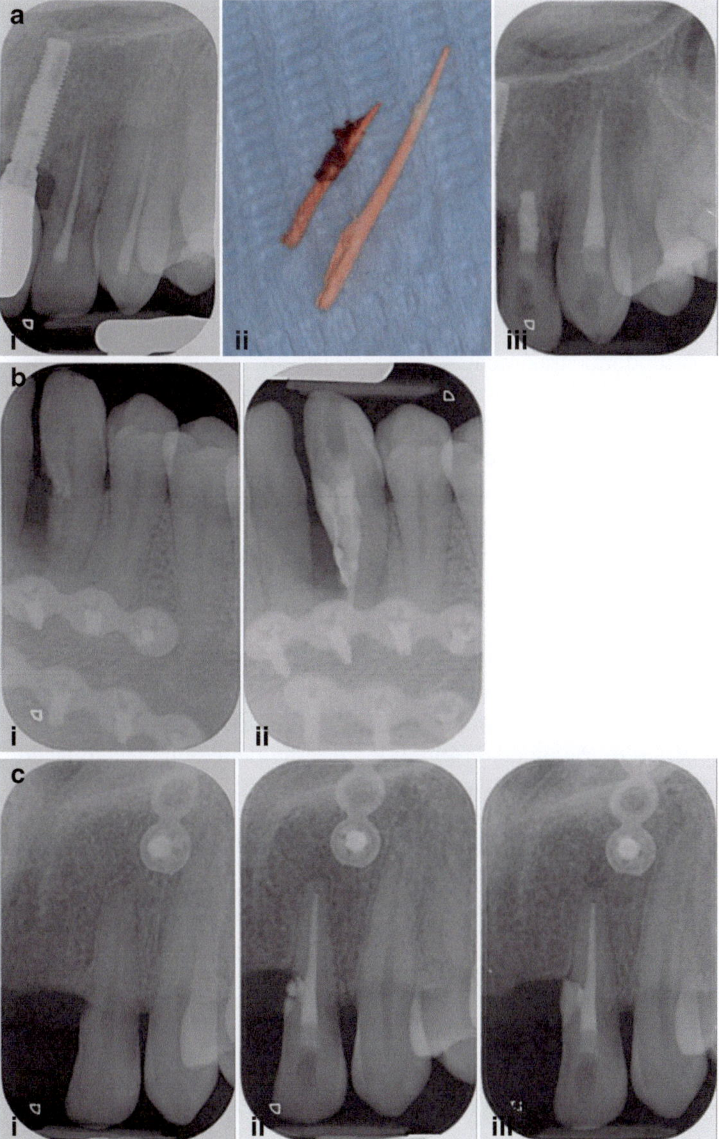

Fig. 2.18 Trauma induced examples of internal and external resorption: In example **a**, the LCPA radiograph of the UL2 shows replacement resorption, with the loss of periodontal ligament space and both the UL23 have developed internal root resorption (i). The photograph (ii) shows the gutta percha (GP) removed from the canals of the UL23 during endodontic re-treatment. The post-operative radiograph shows internal and external resorption in the UL2, and internal resorption in the UL3 (iii). In example **b** ((i) LCPA radiograph of the LL3 pre-operatively, and (ii) LCPA radiograph of the LL3 post-operatively) internal and external resorption of the LL3 has been treated non-surgically and surgically respectively. In example **c** ((i) pre-operative LCPA radiograph of the UL2, (ii) LCPA radiograph of the UL2 post-root canal treatment and (iii) LCPA radiograph of the UL2, post-surgical repair of the mesial external resorption defect) resorption communicating with the periodontal and endodontic structures has been treated. Both examples **b** and **c** show that the periodontal architecture re-established below the level of the repaired resorption defects

endodontic treatment (Yoshpe et al. 2020). A periodontal treatment procedure where the protective layer of cementum is removed does not seem to lead to replacement resorption. Surface resorption results form injury to the root surface (mechanical via trauma or pressure, or chemical due to microbes) and may be self-arresting if the insult stops, with repaired surface made of cementoid tissue (Andreasen 1985).

Invasive, or sometimes called cervical resorption is as a result of invasion from cells of the periodontal ligament and is only symptomatic if there is pulpal or periodontal infection. Susceptibility to cervical resorption is thought to be due to absence of uncalcified pre-cementum or reduced enamel epithelium (Southman 1967), however, the aetiology is not fully understood (Lin et al. 2022). There are some thoughts that trauma, parafunction, poor oral hygiene, periodontal infection, extraction of adjacent teeth, orthodontic treatment, periodontal treatment and internal bleaching of teeth may predispose to cervical resorption (Lin et al. 2022). In the late stages of invasive/cervical resorption, the enamel may be undermined by the growing soft tissue, giving a pink hue to the tooth. There may be involvement of the pulp, the gingival sulcus, persistent inflammation of the periodontium adjacent to the resorption site, with increased pocket depth and pus discharge during probing or presence of pulpal necrosis (Rotstein and Simon 2004). Sometimes the relationship between external and internal resorption is only visible after completion of endodontic treatment (Case 5).

Case 5 The diagnosis between internal and external resorption may be more evident after endodontic treatment (Fig. 2.19a, b). In this case a periodontal pocket of 3 mm remained despite good oral hygiene being established, as the resorption is at the cervical level and crest of bone. Surgical repair may reduce the periodontal pocket through recession. The patient opted to continue with supportive periodontal care rather than carry out surgical repair (Fig. 2.19c).

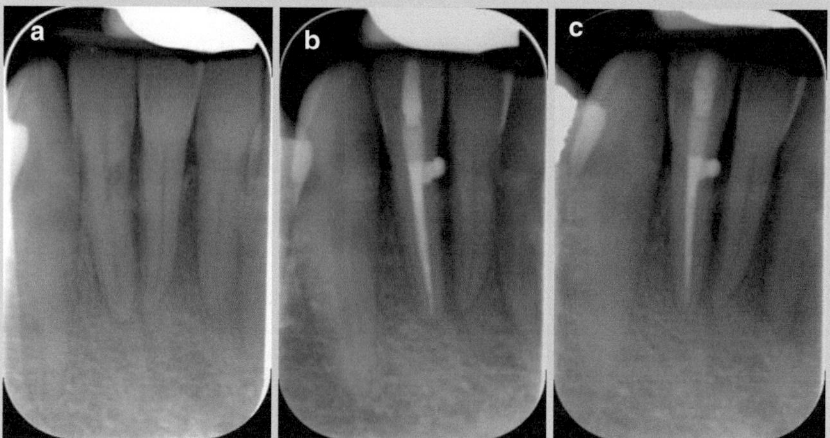

Fig. 2.19 LCPA radiograph of the LR2 (**a**) pre-operatively, (**b**) following completion of root canal treatment in 2017 and (**c**) I year follow-up in 2018

In some cases, there may well be pulpal necrosis, however, due to the reaction of the pulp to surgical exploration and repair, calcification or blockage of the canal during surgical repair, may lead to inability in locating the canal system. Eventually this may lead to the development of a periapical lesion (Case 6 and 7). The tooth may remain without periodontal involvement, however in time, the untreated periapical lesion may lead to a perio-endo lesion in periodontally susceptible patients. External resorption can also be associated with some level of bone loss, seen as a vertical bone defect on the radiographs, extending to the most apical aspect of the resorptive defect (Fig. 2.18b, c, Case 5, Case 8).

Case 6 32-year old patient with cervical resorption of the LL3 (Fig. 2.20a), treated with surgical exploration and repair (Fig. 2.20b), where predentine over the pulp space was visible during surgery. The tooth remains asymptomatic, with positive tests to sensibility testing and without development of apical pathology (Fig. 2.20c).

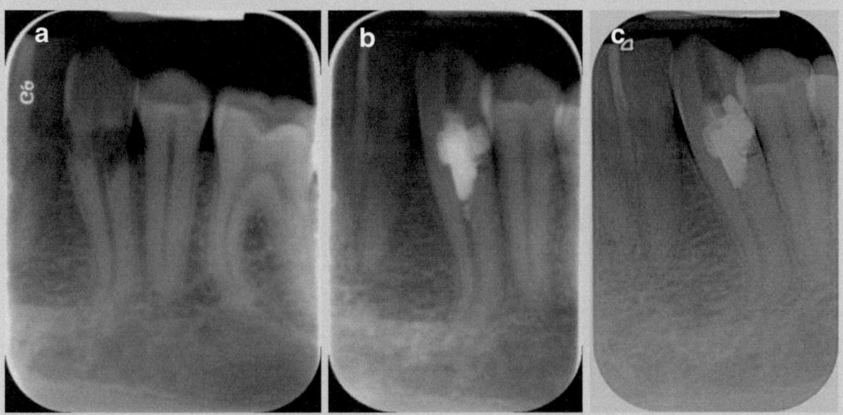

Fig. 2.20 LCPA radiograph of the LL3 (**a**) pre-operatively revealing a disto-cervical radiolucency associated with the LL3 in 2018, without associated peri-apical pathology, (**b**) post-surgical exploration and repair in 2018 and (**c**) at review in 2021

Case 7 A 75-year-old male presented with a lingual cervical resorption defect associated with the LL5 (Fig. 2.21a, b). Due to being asymptomatic and positive to sensibility testing without signs of infection, the patient initially opted to monitor the LL5 (Fig. 2.22a, b), and eventually agreed to surgically explore and repair the resorption defect. During surgical exploration the predentine around the pulp chamber was visible, and therefore, the defect was repaired, and root canal treatment was not instigated (Fig. 2.23a, b). At the

18 month review the resorption defect appeared to have extended more apically, with a possible development of periapical radiolucency. Attempts to find the canal system were futile due to sclerosis of the canal system with no bleeding seen within the canal. What could be instrumented was filled with MTA (Fig. 2.24a). The patient remains asymptomatic, with no tenderness to percussion or other signs of infection, although the apical area appears to be larger on the radiograph (Fig. 2.24b).

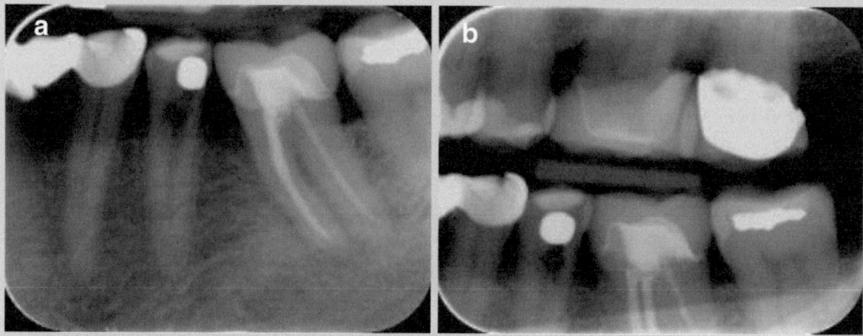

Fig. 2.21 (**a**) LCPA radiograph and (**b**) left bitewing radiograph revealing the presence of a resorptive defect in the LL5 (Aug 2018)

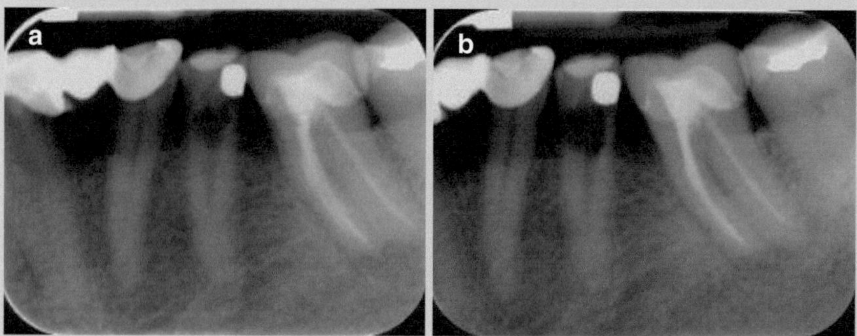

Fig. 2.22 (**a**) LCPA radiograph of the LL5 in Dec 2018 and (**b**) LCPA radiograph of the LL5 in June 2019

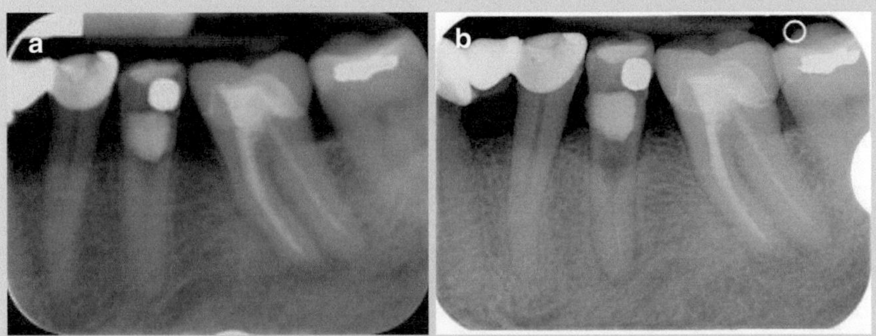

Fig. 2.23 (**a**) LCPA radiograph of the LL5 following surgical repair of the resorption defect (June 2019) and (**b**) LCPA radiograph of the LL5 at follow up in Dec 2020 showing progression of the resorptive defect with possible widening of the periodontal ligament, not yet the development of a periapical radiolucency

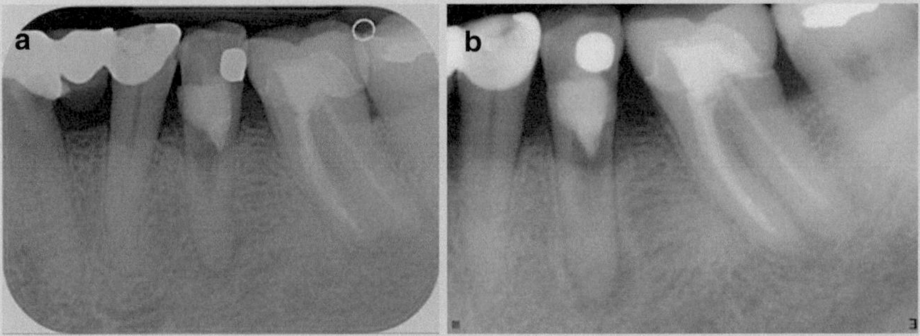

Fig. 2.24 (**a**) LCPA radiograph of the LL5 (Feb 2021) following root canal treatment and obturation of what could be instrumented of the canal system, and (**b**) follow up radiograph (Nov 2021) showing progression of the apical radiolucency and the resorptive defect

Case 8 A 20-year-old female presented with an external cervical resorption defect associated with the LR3. The only history of trauma was orthodontic treatment. The tooth was always slightly sensitive to brush, and positive to sensibility testing without signs of infection (plain film (Fig. 2.25a) and CBCT images 2018 (Fig. 2.26a–e)). The resorptive lesion was repaired surgically (Fig. 2.25b, c). The LR3 continued to test positive to sensibility testing without tenderness to percussion. Despite evidence of communication with the periodontal tissues, a periodontal pocket was not seen clinically. The resorptive lesion has continued slowly despite attempted repair, and bone levels have re-established below the level of resorptive lesion (Fig. 2.27a–d). Calculus was seen adjacent to the resorptive defect (this irritation may contribute to further resorption).

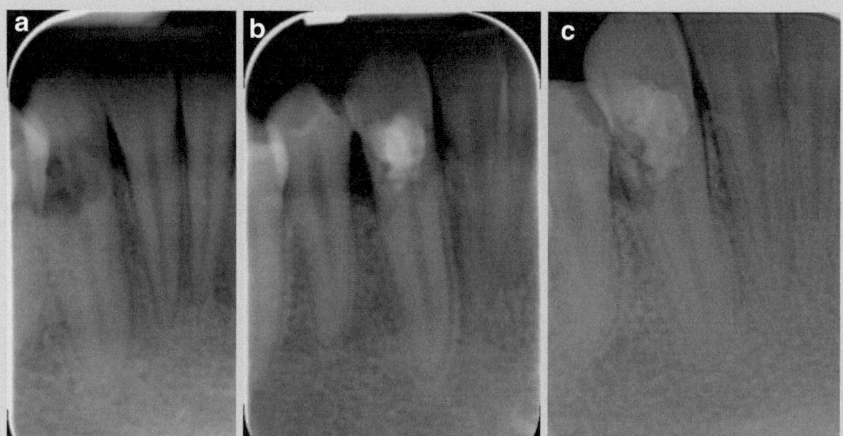

Fig. 2.25 (**a**) LCPA radiograph of the LR3 revealing the presence of a resorptive defect in the cervical region of the LR3 (2018), (**b**) LCPA radiograph of the LL3 following surgical exploration and repair (2019) and (**c**) LCPA radiograph of the LR3 showing progression of the resorptive defect without development of a periapical radiolucency

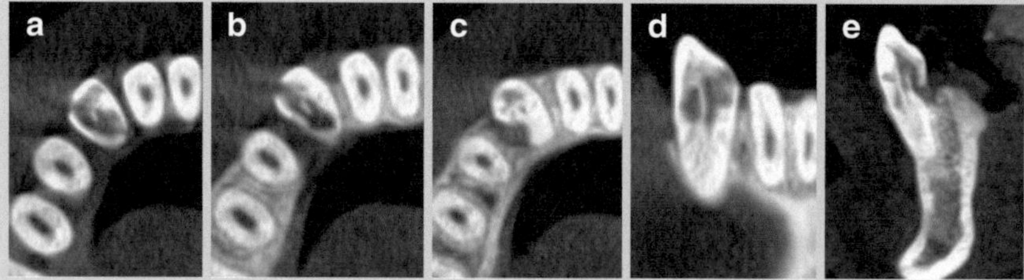

Fig. 2.26 CBCT images (2018) of the LR3: (**a, b** and **c**) Axial CBCT images show the presence of external invasive resorption associated with the LR3 in the coronal half of the tooth. (**d**) Sagittal CBCT image shows the dentine around the pulp chamber, which indicates that this is not internal resorption and has not yet involved the pulp tissue. (**e**) Sagittal CBCT image shows the distolingual bone level below the apical extent of the resorptive lesion

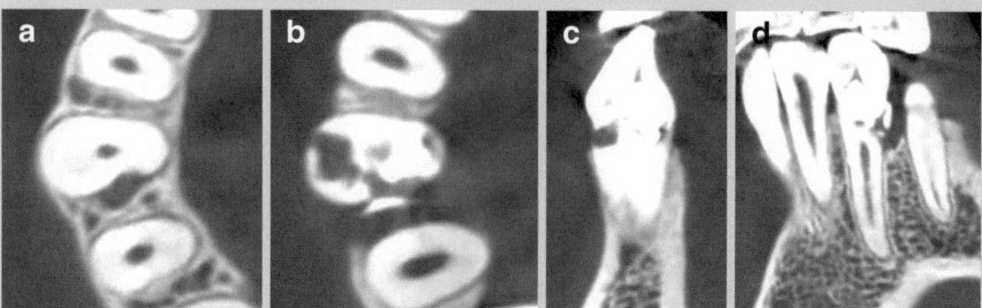

Fig. 2.27 CBCT images (2023) of the LR3: (**a**) Axial CBCT image after repair of the resorptive defect shows distal radiolucency within the bone remained unchanged from 2018. (**b**) Axial CBCT image shows the surgical repair wrapping around the canal system. (**c**) Sagittal CBCT image of the LR3 revealed perforation of the buccal cervical dentine. (**d**) Coronal CBCT image shows the bone levels on the distolingual aspect having established below the resorptive defect and repair, in this patient who is not periodontally susceptible

There are many classifications of resorption defects (Lin et al. 2022), and most recently a new classification taking into consideration anatomical, physiological, pathological and aetiological aspects has been published (Abbott and Lin 2022). Tooth and root resorption have been classified into internal or external, with a number of subtypes (Table 2.2). More than one type of resorption could be happening in the same tooth.

Table 2.2 Classification of tooth resorption (Abbott and Lin 2022)

	Surface resorption	Inflammatory resorption	Replacement resorption	Other
Internal (begins within the pulp or dentine and moves towards the PDL)	1. Internal surface resorption Small superficial areas of the dentine walls affected, transient and self-limiting. Due to transient irritation of the pulp (e.g. trauma or external bleaching) or just before pulp becomes necrotic (due to caries or cracks, leaking restorations). Not easy to see radiographically.	2. Internal inflammatory resorption Continued entry of bacteria from trauma, caries or cracks leads to inflammation or necrosis coronal to the resorptive defect. Pulp replaced by periodontal like connective tissue. Resorptive area contains dentinoclasts and granulation tissue. Occasionally present with pulpitic pain.	3. Internal replacement resorption Rare condition when dentine and pulp replaced by bone. Due to trauma or insult to pulp. Pink discolouration, asymptomatic and may or may not respond to sensibility testing. Radiographically seen as mixed radiolucent and radiopaque areas in pulp space.	
External (begins in the cementum or outer dentine and moves towards the pulp)	1. External surface resorption Transient, reaction to minor trauma, superficial and on cementum of root surfaces. Only progresses if the root contaminated with bacteria.	2. External inflammatory resorption which may be (a) apical or (b) lateral Usually due to traumatic injuries that damage the cementum/PDL cells (luxation, avulsion) as well as necrosis of the pulp chamber through bacterial contamination. Can be symptomatic of apical periodontitis. Loss of lamina dura at the site of resorption and irregular root shape.	3. External replacement resorption which may be (a) transient or (b) progressive Cementum and dentine replaced by bone. If ankylosed, a high-pitched, metallic sound may be heard on percussion, often without obvious mobility of the tooth. Radiographically, the lack of lamina dura and PDL space is seen, with bone adjacent to dentine.	4. External invasive resorption – starts in a subgingival location and can spread in all directions. 5. External pressure resorption – resorption as a result of pressure of adjacent tooth, tumour, or cyst. 6. Orthodontic resorption – shortened roots of one or more teeth following orthodontic treatment, asymptomatic and usually root apices affected. 7. Physiological resorption – process by which primary teeth exfoliate, slow process if secondary successor not present. 8. Idiopathic resorption – rare and without any other stimulation which may cause resorption, usually involves multiple teeth, and may have contributing medical history.

Internal resorption can be superficial and termed 'surface', however, if the insult remains, can become inflammatory. In both situations the odontoblasts and pre-dentine are lost to varying degrees. In inflammatory internal resorption, the tissue apical to the resorptive defect will be inflamed when the resorption is active, but will eventually become necrotic, resulting in arrest of the resorption. If the pulp space is infected, apical periodontitis will develop. In the rare occurrence of replacement resorption, root canal treatment may not be possible or required. The tooth may sound ankylosed, and only requires monitoring.

External resorption can also be classified into 'surface' (self-limiting and does not require any treatment), 'inflammatory' (has an infected canal and the root surface has been damaged) or 'replacement' (cementum and periodontal ligament cells damaged, leading to bone/root resorption and bone deposition). External inflammatory resorption can occur if there is communication between the root canal system and the peri-radicular tissues (exit of main or lateral canals) as there can be escape of microbes and their endotoxins from the root canal system. Long standing endodontic infections due to deep periodontal pockets, cracks within the tooth/root, leaking restorations can also lead to external inflammatory resorption. Root canal treatment in teeth with mature roots, and potentially regeneration in teeth with immature roots may be considered, often after medicating the canal to stabilise the resorption process. Many forms of external resorption may lead to ankylosis, however ankylosis can occur without the presence of resorption. The loss of the periodontal ligament (PDL) space and associated cells may lead to resorption at the site of ankylosis. External invasive resorption may develop where cementum is damaged by repeated periodontal treatment, with some patients describing an altered sensation when brushing their teeth. The lesion may be found with periodontal probing, with some degree of reduced mobility of the tooth, if ankylosed. Radiographically, an irregularly shaped radiolucency with ectopic bone-like tissue may be seen (Heithersay 1999). Treatment may include periodontal surgery and endodontic treatment, without guarantee of arresting the resorptive process. In some cases, it may be more appropriate to monitor such teeth, until problematic, and then extract (Case 9). External pressure resorption may mimic symptoms of apical periodontitis or periodontal disease, such as tenderness to percussion or mobility. Orthodontic resorption is often seen to shorten or blunt the apices of teeth without pulpal involvement or loss of PDL space. In periodontally susceptible patient, this may lead to further mobility of periodontally involved teeth.

Case 9 Orthodontic treatment and periodontal susceptibility can lead to both bone loss and resorption. A 44-year old asymptomatic patient presented having been diagnosed and treated for periodontal disease at the age of 18 years and also underwent 2 years of fixed orthodontic treatment. Medically, the patient was a fit and well, a life-long non-smoker, without known drug allergies or regular medication. In 2018 (Fig. 2.28), there were periodontal pockets of

5–6 mm, which resolved with improvement in oral hygiene and non-surgical periodontal treatment. At review in 2023 (Fig. 2.29), there were no deep pockets, bleeding on probing or suppuration. There were no clinical signs of apical periodontitis and a number of teeth had been splinted together by her general dental practitioner. The progression of the periodontal disease may be slow, with periodontal treatment in a well-motivated patient. Due to the level of root resorption, endodontic involvement may be inevitable in the presence of periodontal inflammation. This slow rate of progression in a well-motivated patient shows the difficulty in making prognostic decisions: most would consider many of these teeth to be of poor prognosis, however the patient was very clear that she would like to maintain these teeth and resisted extraction for many decades.

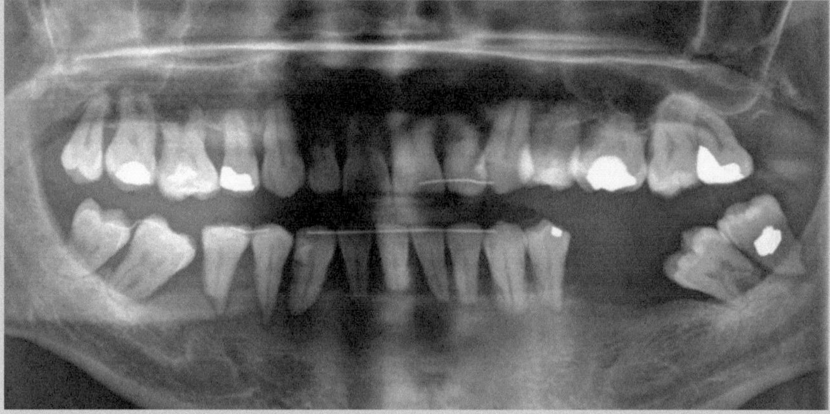

Fig. 2.28 DPT showing generalised horizontal bone loss and severe resorption of the roots of almost all teeth in 2018

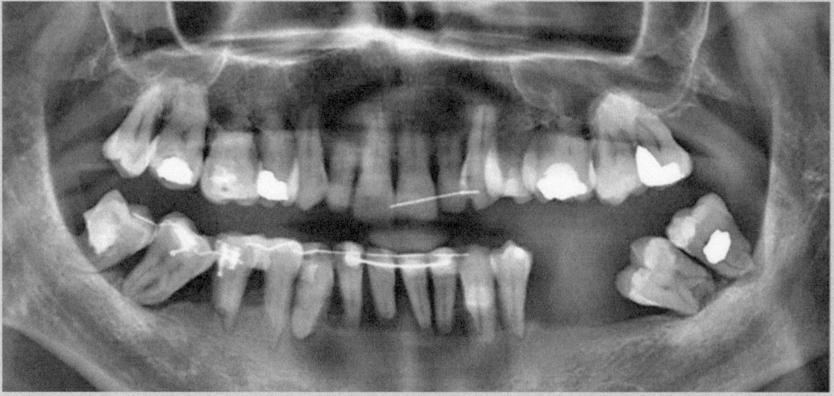

Fig. 2.29 DPT showing no significant change in the level of generalised horizontal bone loss and severe resorption of the roots in 2023

References

Abbott PV, Lin S. Tooth resorption-Part 2: a clinical classification. Dent Traumatol. 2022;38(4):267–85.

Abbott PV, Salgado JC. Strategies for the endodontic management of concurrent endodontic and periodontal diseases. Aust Dent J. 2009;54:S70–85.

Adriaens PA, De Boever JA, Loesche WJ. Bacterial invasion in root cementum and radicular dentin of periodontally diseased teeth in humans. A reservoir of periodontopathic bacteria. J Periodontol. 1988;59:222–30.

Ahmed HMA, Hashem AA. Accessory roots and root canals in human anterior teeth: a review and clinical considerations. Int Endod J. 2016;49:724–36.

Anand V, Govila V, Gulati M. Endo-perio lesion: part i (the pathogenesis) – a review. Arch Dental Sci. 2012;3(1):3–9.

Andreasen JO. External root resorption: its implication in dental traumatology, paedodontics, periodontics, orthodontics and endodontics. Int Endod J. 1985;18:109–18.

Aryanpour S, Bercy P, Van Nieuwenhuysen JP. Endodontic and periodontal treatments of a geminated mandibular first premolar. Int Endod J. 2002;35:209–124.

Bender IB, Seltzer S. The effect of periodontal disease on the pulp. Oral Surg Oral Med Oral Pathol. 1972;33:458–74.

Bennett DT, Miles AE. Observations on the permeability of human calcified dental tissues to penicillin. J Dent Res. 1955;34:553–62.

Bergenholtz G. Micro-organisms from necrotic pulp of traumatised teeth. Odontol Rev. 1974;25:347–58.

Bergenholtz G, Lindhe J. Effect of experimentally induced marginal periodontitis and periodontal scaling on the dental pulp. J Clin Periodontol. 1978;5:59–73.

Carranza F, Newman M, Takei H. Carranza's clinical periodontology. 10th ed. St. Louis: Elsevier Saunders; 2006.

Carrigan PJ, Morse DR, Furst ML, Sinai IH. A scanning electron microscopic evaluation of human dentinal tubules according to age and location. J Endod. 1984;10:359–63.

Chapple ILC, Lumley PJ. The perio-endo interface. Dent Update. 1999;26:331–41.

Clauder T, Shin SJ. Repair of perforations with MTA: clinical actions and mechanisms of action. Endod Topics. 2009;15:32–55.

Czarnecki RT, Schilder H. A histological evaluation of the human pulp in teeth with varying degrees of periodontal disease. J Endod. 1979;5(8):242–52.

Dongari A, Lambrianidis T. Periodontally derived pulpal lesions. Endod Dent Traumatol. 1988;4:49–54.

Dummer PM, McGinn JH, Rees DG. The position and topography of the apical canal constriction and apical foramen. Int Endod J. 1984;17(4):192–8.

Farzaneh M, Abitbol S, Friedman S. Treatment outcome in endodontics: the Toronto study. Phases I and II: orthograde retreatment. J Endod. 2004;30(9):627–33.

Fulari SG, Tambake DP. Rootless teeth: dentin dysplasia type I. Contemp Clin Dent. 2013;4(4):520–2.

Furseth R. The fine structure of acellular cementum in young human premolars. Scand J Dent Res. 1974;82:437–41.

Fuss Z, Tsesis I, Lin S. Root resorption–diagnosis, classification and treatment choices based on stimulation factors. Dent Traumatol. 2003;19:175–82.

Gordon MPJ, Chandler NP. Electronic apex locators. Int Endod J. 2004;37:425–37.

Gu YC. A micro-computed tomographic analysis of. maxillary lateral incisors with radicular grooves. J Endod. 2011;37(6):789–92.

Gutman JL. Prevalence, location and patency of accessory canals in the furcation region of permanent molars. J Periodontol. 1978;49:21.

Hanisch M, Bohner L, Sabandal MMI, et al. Oral symptoms and oral health-related quality of life of individuals with x-linked hypophosphatemia. Head Face Med. 2019;15:8.

Hansen EK, Asmussen E. Cusp fracture of endodontically treated posterior teeth restored with amalgam: Teeth restored in Denmark before 1975 versus after 1979. Acta Odontol Scand. 1993;51:73–7.

Hargreaves KM, Cohen S, Berman LH. Cohen's pathways of the pulp. 10th ed. St. Louis: Mosby Elsevier; 2011.

Heithersay GS. Clinical, radiologic, and histopathologic features of invasive cervical resorption. Quintessence Int. 1999;30:27–37.

Hülsmann M, Bahr R, Grohmann U. Hemisection and vital treatment of a fused tooth—literature review and case report. Endod Dent Traumatol. 1997;13:253–8.

Jeng P-Y, Pitarch ALLRM, Chang M-C, Wu Y-H, Jeng J-H. Cemental tear: to know what we have neglected in dental practice. J Formos Med Assoc. 2018;117(4):261–7.

Kakoli P, Nandakumar R, Romberg E, Arola D, Fouad AF. The effect of age on bacterial penetration of radicular dentin. J Endod. 2009;35:78–81.

Keskin C, Güler DH. A retrospective study of the prevalence of cemental tear in a sample of the adult population applied ondokuz mayis university faculty of dentistry. Meandros Med Dent J. 2017;18:115–9.

Kim HJ, Choi Y, Yu MK, Lee KW, Min KS. Recognition and management of palatogingival groove for tooth survival: a literature review. Restor Dent Endod. 2017;42(2):77–86.

Kishen A. Mechanisms and risk factors for fracture predilection in endodontically treated teeth. Endod Top. 2006;13:57–83.

Kuttler Y. Microscopic investigation of root apexes. J Am Dent Assoc. 1955;50:544–52.

Langeland K, Rodrigues H, Dowden W. Periodontal disease, bacteria, and pulpal histopathology. Oral Surg Oral Med Oral Pathol. 1974;37:257–70.

Lantelme RL, Handelman SL, Herbison RJ. Dentin formation in periodontally diseased teeth. J Dent Res. 1976;55:48–51.

Lee BN, Jung HY, Chang HS, Hwang YC, Oh WM. Dental management of patients with X-linked hypophosphatemia. Restor Dent Endod. 2017;42(2):146–51.

Lin HJ, Chan CP, Yang CY, Wu CT, Tsai YL, Huang CC, Yang KD, Lin CC, Chang SH, Jeng JH. Cemental tear: clinical characteristics and its predisposing factors. J Endod. 2011;37(5):611–8.

Lin HJ, Chang SH, Chang MC, Tsai YL, Chiang CP, Chan CP, Jeng JH. Clinical fracture site, morphologic and histopathologic characteristics of cemental tear: role in endodontic lesions. J Endod. 2012;38(8):1058–62.

Lin HJ, Chang MC, Chang SH, Wu CT, Tsai YL, Huang CC, Chang SF, Cheng YW, Chan CP, Jeng JH. Treatment outcome of the teeth with cemental tears. J Endod. 2014;40(9):1315–20.

Lin S, Moreinos D, Kaufman AY, Abbott PV. Tooth resorption – part 1: the evolvement, rationales and controversies of tooth resorption. Dent Traumatol. 2022;38(4):253–66.

Lindhe J, Lang NP, Karring T. Clinical periodontology and implant dentistry. Oxford: Blackwell Munksgaard; 2008.

Mondelli J, Steagall L, Ishikiriama A, de Lima Navarro MF, Soares FB. Fracture strength of human teeth with cavity preparations. J Prosthet Dent. 1980;43(4):419–22.

Nanci A. Ten Cate's oral histology development, structure and function. 7th ed. St. Louis: Mosby; 2008. p. 210–1.

Nanci A, Bosshardt DD. Structure of the periodontal tissues in health and disease. Periodontology. 2006;40:11–28.

Ong TK, Harun N, Lim TW. Cemental tear on maxillary anterior incisors: a description of clinical, radiographic, and histopathological features of two clinical cases. Eur Endod J. 2019;4:90–5.

Petelin M, Skaleric U, Cevc P, Schara M. The permeability of human cementum in vitro measured by electron paramagnetic resonance. Arch Oral Biol. 1999;44:259–67.

Pitts DL, Matheny HE, Nicholls JI. An in vitro study of spreader loads required to cause vertical root fracture during lateral condensation. J Endod. 1983;9(12):544–50.

Randow K, Glantz PO. On cantilever loading of vital and non-vital teeth. An experimental clinical study. Acta Odontol Scand. 1986;44:271–47.

Ravanshad S, Khayat A. Endodontic therapy on a dentition exhibiting multiple periapical radiolucencies associated with dentinal dysplasia type 1. Aust Endod J. 2006;32(1):40–2.

Reeh ES, Messer HH, Douglas WH. Reduction in tooth stiffness as a result of endodontic and restorative procedures. J Endod. 1989;15(11):512–6.

Ricucci D. Apical limit of root canal instrumentation and obturation, part 1. Literature review. Int Endod J. 1998;31(6):384–93.

Ricucci D, Langeland K. Apical limit of root canal instrumentation and obturation, part 2. A histological study. Int Endod J. 1998;31(6):394–409.

Ricucci D, Siqueira JF Jr. Fate of the tissue in lateral canals and apical ramifications in response to pathologic conditions and treatment procedures. J Endod. 2010;36:1–15.

Riffle AB. Dentine: it's physical characteristics during curettage. J Periodontol. 1953;24:232–41.

Rotstein I, Simon JH. Diagnosis, prognosis and decision-making in the treatment of combined periodontal-endodontic lesions. Periodontol 2000. 2004;34:165–203.

Rubach WC, Mitchell DF. Periodontal disease, accessory canals and pulp pathosis. J Periodontol. 1964;36:34–8.

Schmidt JC, Sahrmann P, Weiger R, Schmidlin PR, Walter C. Biologic width dimensions--a systematic review. J Clin Periodontol. 2013;40(5):493–504.

Seltzer S, Bender IB, Ziontz M. The dynamics of pulp inflammation: correlations between diagnostic data and actual histologic findings in the pulp. Oral Surg Oral Med Oral Pathol. 1963a;16:969–77.

Seltzer S, Bender IB, Ziontz M. The interrelationship of pulp and periodontal disease. Oral Surg Oral Med Oral Pathol. 1963b;16:1474.

Seltzer S, Bender IB, Nazimov H, Sinai I. Pulpitis induced interradicular periodontal change in experimental animals. J Periodontol. 1967;38:124.

Seow WK. Developmental defects of enamel and dentine: challenges for basic science research and clinical management. Aus Dent J. 2014;59(1):143–54.

Simon JH, Glick DH, Frank AL. Predictable endodontic and periodontic failure as a result of radicular anomalies. Oral Surg Oral Med Oral Pathol. 1971;31:823–6.

Somerman MJ, Morrison GM, Alexander MB, Foster RA. Structure and composition of cementum. In: Bowen W, Tabak L, editors. Cariology of the Nineteenninetees. New York: U. Rochester Press; 1993. p. 155–71.

Southman J. Clinical and histological aspects of peripheral cervical resorption. J Periodontool. 1967;38:534–8.

Stein TJ, Corcoran JF. Anatomy of the root apex and its histologic changes with age. Oral Surg Oral Med Oral Pathol. 1990;69:238–42.

Tagger M. Tooth germination treated by endodontic therapy. J Endod. 1975;1:181–4.

Thomas RP. Root canal morphology of maxillary permanent first molar teeth at various ages [Masters Thesis]. University of Sydney, 1986.

Tammaro S, Wennström JL, Bergenholtz G. Root-dentin sensitivity following non-surgical periodontal treatment. J Clin Periodontol. 2000;27(9):690–7.

Trabert KC, Caput AA, Abou-Rass M. Tooth fracture: a comparison of endodontic and restorative treatments. J Endod. 1978;4(11):341–5.

Tronstad L. Root resorption — etiology, terminology and clinical manifestations. Dent Traumatol. 1988;4(6):241–52.

Trope M, Ray HL. Resistance to fracture of endodontically treated roots. Oral Surg Oral Med Oral Pathol. 1992;73:99–102.

Wassermann F, Blayney JR, Groetzinger G, DeWitt TG. Studies on the different pathways of exchange of minerals in teeth with the aid of radioactive phosphorus. J Dent Res. 1941;20:389–98.

Whyman RA. Endodontic-periodontic lesions. Part 1; prevalence, aetiology and diagnosis. N Z Dent J. 1988;84:74.

Yoshpe M, Einy S, Ruparel N, Lin S, Kaufman AY. Regenerative end- odontics: a potential solution for external root resorption (case series). J Endod. 2020;46:192–9.

Zehnder M, Gold SI, Hasselgren G. Pathologic interaction in pulpal and periodontal tissues. J Clin Periodontol. 2002;29:663–71.

Periodontal and Endodontic Pathogens

Abstract

The following chapter is an introduction to the pathogens that reside within the periodontal and endodontic structures. It is not an exhaustive list of microbes or their behaviour; however aims to provide an overview of the complexity of the oral microbiota.

Microbes in Health

In health, there are over 600 species of micro-organisms within the oral cavity (Moore and Moore 1994; Curtis et al. 2020; Feng and Weinberg 2006). Some of the microbes are good, only some are bad, some we have yet to discover, some have not yet been cultured successfully and some live in a biofilm that is hard to penetrate. Many are present in health and disease. Bacterial species considered to be 'good', such as *Streptococcus sanguis*, *Streptococcus mitis*, *Actinomyces naeslundii* and *Actinomyces viscosus*, may prevent colonization of more pathogenic bacteria and may even kill opportunistic pathogens. Others, such as *Prevotella intermedia*, *Porphyromonas gingivalis*, *Aggregatibacter (formally Actinobacillus) actinomycetemcomitans*, may be considered 'bad' because they lead to pathological consequences.

Commensal organisms live in the oral cavity, in some cases deriving nutrients from their neighbours, without damaging these neighbours, and in other cases competing with others to establish micro-niches. Commensal organisms tend not to activate the host's immune system (Feng and Weinberg 2006). Many microbes are likely to live in a biofilm where there is sharing of Deoxyribonucleic Acid (DNA), quorum sensing and 'learning from their neighbours' to change from good to bad and vice versa. Quorum sensing allows communication between bacteria to control specific factors such as the formation of biofilms and virulence factor expression, which are tightly controlled and influenced by environmental changes. When pathogenic bacteria cause permeability of the epithelium, commensal bacteria can also enter the underlying connective tissue and contribute to inflammation (Feng and Weinberg 2006). Microbiota is complex and dynamic, and exist in a perpetually changing local environment with host mediated selective pressures. Microbiota is a hard to study biofilm and only 50–60% of the subgingival microbiota can be grown in a laboratory.

A biofilm is a community of micro-organisms adhered to a surface, and is polymicrobial. Microbes may be competing with each other, but equally may be helping and protecting each other. Biofilms are thought to grow like tall buildings with some channels and spaces in between them. These channels house hydrocolloid matrix of polymers and lots of DNA, also creating environmental gradients (nutrients, oxygen, pH, metabolic products) where microbes can share nutrients and DNA. Molecules can take time to diffuse through the hydrocolloid, and larger molecules like antibiotics, may not be able to pass deep into the biofilm.

Pathogens in Periodontal Lesions

Subgingival dental plaque contains 415 of the 600 species of micro-organisms found in the oral cavity (Feng and Weinberg 2006), where as the healthy dental pulp is a sterile structure. There is a difficulty in providing evidence for 'causation' of one microbial group in periodontal destruction, as introduction of these microbes into healthy animals does not necessarily cause the disease. Knowledge of microbiota is evolving with technology and is incomplete. A diverse consortium of micro-organisms that are part of the endogenous microbiota of most people can cause periodontal breakdown only for some (Feng and Weinberg 2006). Many of the suspects represent 1–5% of the colony forming units at sites with chronic periodontitis. It is possible that there is a complex relationship between the oral microbiota and the host response, leading to periodontal destruction. However, some of the key information that is known is described below.

Components of saliva, gingival crevicular fluid, bacterial and host cell debris form the dental pellicle, which is the first stage of the development of plaque. The pellicle on non-shedding hard tissue is a substrate for the accumulation of bacteria. The microbes found in plaque differ in the plaque closest to the tooth surface (mainly gram positive cocci and rods) from that facing the oral cavity (mainly gram negative rods, filaments and spirochetes). Additionally, there is a difference in supragingival and subgingival plaque. Subgingival plaque houses more anaerobic bacteria. Bacteria within subgingival plaque are nourished by a good blood supply, however, this also means a host immune response to influence bacterial colonisation (Carranza et al. 2006). Plaque is a biofilm, which matures with time: the more long-standing the more complex the microbiota. Supragingival plaque also contains mineral from saliva, and with increasing amounts of mineral, plaque calcifies to form calculus. The mineral for subgingival plaque comes from gingival crevicular fluid, and blood products probably contribute to the dark green/brown colour of subgingival calculus. Calculus is likely to be covered by a layer of soft plaque. It is thought that a susceptible host, presence of pathogenic bacteria and absence of beneficial bacteria are required for the development of periodontal disease (Carranza et al. 2006).

Socransky et al. (1998) catergorised the microbial complexes in periodontal disease into five groups: 'Red' (in to which *Porphyromonas gingivalis*, *Treponema denticola, Basteroids forsythus* fall), 'Orange' (in to which *Fusobacterium nucleatum* subspecies and *Prevoltella intermedia* fall), 'Yellow' (streptococci), 'Green' (*Capnocytophagaspeciaes, A. actinomycetemcomitans* Serotype a), and 'Purple' (*Actinomyces odontolyticus, Vaillonella parvula*). Species of the 'red' complex were rarely seen in the absence of those in the 'orange' complex, with species from the red and orange complex being strongly associated with deeper periodontal pockets and those of the red complex being associated with bleeding on probing (Socransky et al. 1998). These red and orange complexes are characterised by their anaerobic Gram-negative virulence factors that maintain an inflammatory response, and have also been found in root canal systems (Sundqvist 1992; Gambin et al. 2021).

'Red' clusters such as *P. gingivalis, T. denticola, Tannerella forsythia,* and *A. actinomycetemcomitans* Serotype b (which did not fall into any of the clusters) are considered more pathogenic because they are not only able to colonise subgingivally, but can adhere and invade tissues, directly modulate chemokine expression in osteoblasts to mediate resorption of bone directly, as well as create proteases and endotoxins that lead to a destructive immune response (Socransky et al. 1998; Feng and Weinberg 2006). *P. gingivalis, Campylobacter rectus, T. forsythia, P. intermedia, Eubacterium* sp, *Parvimonas micra, Treponema* sp. can all be seen in those susceptible to periodontal disease, but can also found in 'periodontitis-resistant' groups. *A. actinomycetemcomitans* has been more often found in those previously described as 'aggressive' cases, however, some with aggressive periodontal disease do not harbour *A. actinomycemcomintans,* whilst also being found in those considered periodontally healthy (Fine et al. 2007; Haubek et al. 2008). Re-emergence of 'red' and 'orange' complexes 3-12 months post debridement is considered to be associated with ongoing loss of attachment at these sites (Haffajee et al. 2006).

The alteration in the micro-organisms from health (gram-positive, facultative, fermentative micro-organisms) towards disease (predominantly gram-negative anaerobic, chemo-organotrophic and proteolytic micro-organisms) leads to an aberrant inflammatory response associated with periodontal breakdown (Haffajee and Socransky 1994; Slots and Taubman 1992; Moore and Moore 1994). In periodontal infections, plaque enhances inflammation and increases the flow of gingival crevicular fluid, thereby increasing the food for certain microbes to out-compete those that are less virulent, and increase the pathogenicity by numerical dominance leading to an increase in proteolytic bacteria at the gingival crevice. It is possible for periodontal microbes to invade cementum and root dentine, with more than 80% of periodontally involved teeth having bacterial within root dentine (Adriaens 1984), penetrating the outer 300 microns of the dentine (Adriaens et al. 1988) making their removal more difficult (Cobb and Sottosanti 2021), especially where there are surface irregularities, micro-fractures and cracks and as well as penetrate cementum. These bacteria and their endotoxins can be reduced but not eliminated by scaling and root planing (Cobb and Sottosanti 2021). Mechanical debridement (root surface debridement and oral hygiene) aims to disrupt the biofilm and change the environment so that this microbial community cannot develop and produce pathogenic products. Professional instrumentation will be disrupting the established plaque biofilm, however, the patient's own oral hygiene will be disrupting the plaque biofilm at least once a day, everyday, preventing maturation to a pathogenic form.

Pathogens in Endodontic Lesions

In endodontics, infection establishes where there previously were no bacteria, and through genetic exchange and mutations, these microbes learn to survive (Sundqvist 1994). In the absence of microbes, it is not possible to develop pulpal and periradicular disease (Kakehashi et al. 1965), and apical bone resorption will only occur if a necrotic pulp becomes infected (Sundqvist 1976; Moller et al. 1981). Some studies have shown that bacteria cannot be cultivated from teeth without apical periodontitis, however, bacteria are always cultivated from teeth with apical periodontitis (Korzen et al. 1974; Sundqvist 1976). Once the pulp is infected, the microbes are within a chamber and with a limited supply of nutrients. Proteolytic bacteria will thrive on the serum influx from periapical inflammation, and flare-ups may occur when the nutrient gradient changes, for example, over instrumentation and enlarging of the apical foramen allows an influx of nutrients from the periapical tissues (Svensater and Bergenholtz 2004).

From the 600 species in the oral cavity, very few establish themselves in the difficult environment of the pulp canal system. Endodontic infections are polymicrobial, with about 10–50 microbial species per infected canal. Due to selective pressures, some microbes thrive where others cannot survive (Paster et al. 2001). Generally, the bacteria within the canal system are strict anaerobes (function at low oxygen-reduction potential and grow only in the absence of oxygen, but vary in their sensitivity to oxygen), obligate anaerobes (lack certain enzymes therefore cannot grow in the presence of oxygen, and may even die in the presence of oxygen), microaerophilic (can grow in the presence of oxygen, but derive most of their energy from anaerobic energy pathways) facultative anaerobes (which can grow in the presence or absence of oxygen,) and in the early stages of necrosis, obligate aerobes (those that require oxygen for growth).

In an untreated canal, the microbes need to breach the enamel, reach the pulp via dentinal tubules, overcome host defenses in the pulp, find nutrition, compete with other micro-organisms, and resist host defenses. Then when the microbes reach the apical portion, they may cause an inflammatory response from the host, which may present as an apical area. The presence of microbes within the apical area is more likely in long standing lesions (Fig. 3.1).

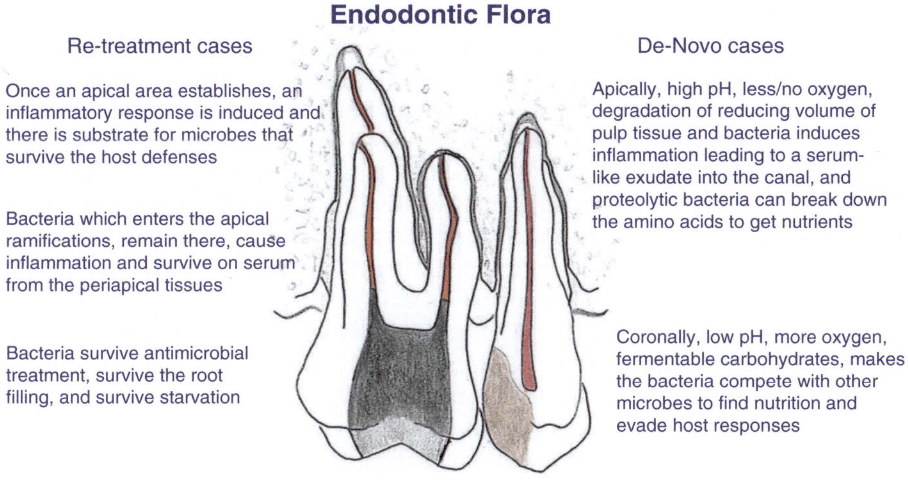

Fig. 3.1 Changes in endodontic flora with time and treatment

The microflora becomes more anaerobic over time (usually 3 months), competing for tissue fluid and necrotic tissue, developing commensal relationships. The nature of the microbes will be determined by the stage of infection, with facultative microbes initially, then most of the microbial flora becoming anaerobic, and teeth with necrotic pulps eventually having 90% strict anaerobic bacteria (Sundqvist 1994). It may take between a few days and up to several years for the whole pulp to become necrotic, depending on the presence and standard of the coronal seal.

In teeth with failed root canal treatment, the microbes would not only have had to survive the initial treatment, but also to survive in an environment of limited nutrition, and by definition be more resilient and resistant to chemo-mechanical debridement (Tronstad and Sunde 2003; Sundqvist and Figdor 2003; Portenier et al. 2003). Microbes can also exist in dentinal tubules, accessory canals, canal ramifications, apical deltas, fins, and transverse anastomoses (Athanassiadis et al. 2007). They can invade dentinal tubules to a depth of between 300 microns and the full length of the tubules to the cementum (Baugh and Wallace 2005). Once a root canal treated tooth has the gutta percha exposed to the oral microbes, the whole canal may be contaminated within 73 days (Torabinejad et al. 1990). It is recommended that endodontic re-treatment be provided for teeth that may have been leaking for more than 3 months (Rotstein and Simon 2004). It must also be borne in mind that all dental materials have a shelf life and use by date, therefore, materials like gutta percha degrade with time and exposure to the oral environment. When access is gained to the gutta percha of failed endodontically treated teeth, it is possible to encounter chalky, degraded gutta percha, often black in colour, with a foul odour as a result of bacterial contamination. The degradation, change in bio-ceramic sealers with time and their ability to maintain a seal is still unknown (Donnermeyer et al. 2019).

There is a correlation between the size of the lesion and amount of bacterial species, with long standing infections and larger lesions having a higher density of bacteria. It has not been possible to differentiate between the microbes that cause a lesion and those that simply reside in the lesions because the environment favours their selection (Zehnder et al. 2002). In heavily infected root canal systems, microbial invasion can vary from a few microns up to half way to the cementodentinal junction, where alteration of the cementum can be observed (Armitage et al. 1983). In acute apical infections, microbes can be found in the periapical tissues, however, in chronic non-symptomatic periapical lesions, endodontic infections cause an inflammatory reaction in the periapical tissues that is free of microbes. Although, polymicrobial infections can spread from the canal to periapical tissues, this is rare as chronic symptomless apical periodontitis lesions are separated from the periapical tissue by a dense wall of polymorphonuclear leukocytes and/or epithelial cells at the apical foramen (Nair 1987). The presence of a draining sinus may indicate the existence of extra radicular infection. Apical areas with suppuration (likely to house microbes beyond the root apex) do still heal after endodontic treatment, with the elimination of the necrotic tissue and granulation tissue followed by regeneration, including periodontal ligament cells migrating to the damaged area, bone regeneration and development of Sharpey's fibres from the periodontal ligament to the bone.

Compared to the same organism in planktonic form (floating in a body of fluid), bacteria within a biofilm (communities encapsulated within a self-developed polymeric matrix, structured and adherent to root surfaces) are 1000× more resistant to antimicrobial agents (Wilson 1996; Costerton and Stewart 2000; Mah and O'Toole 2001; Svensater and Bergenholtz 2004). There is a host response; therefore, some say that the apical area is an area that bacteria are 'killed in' rather than an area for bacteria to 'grow in', although bacteria can invade periapical tissues to cause an extra-radicular infection (Tronstad and Sunde 2003).

Microbiology within periodontal pockets is usually rods and motile organisms, and those within an infected root canal system are rods and cocci (Peeran et al. 2013). Some have suggested that the bacteria within an endodontic infection are very similar to the bacteria found in a periodontal pocket with active disease, however the ratio of anaerobes is 100× higher in a root canal (Rupf et al. 2000; Tronstad and Sunde 2003; Sundqvist and Figdor 2003). Some bacteria, such as *Porphyromonas endodontalis*, are only found in endodontic lesions (van Winkelhoff et al. 1988). Some microbes, such as *Enterococcus faecalis*, are survivors and found in failed cases of endodontics, able to survive treatment and starvation for extended periods of time (Portenier et al. 2003; Siqueira and Rocas 2004).

Pathogens in Perio-Endo Lesions

In periodontal and endodontic disease, the pathogens are eventually mainly of an anaerobic nature, with similar microflora being found in deep pockets and adjacent necrotic pulps (Zehnder et al. 2002; Herrera et al. 2018). It must be noted that periodontal lesions contain dense cells, host response and a blood supply, and endodontic lesions have no blood supply, and therefore, tend to be more anaerobic. It has been shown that the flora of endodontic infections is similar to that in periodontal pockets of patients with active periodontal disease (Tronstad and Sunde 2003; Nair 1987; Rupf et al. 2000).

Some have shown that periodontal pathogens accompany endodontic infections with samples from combined perio-endo lesions showing the presence of *A. actinomycemtecomitans*, *F. nucleatum*, *Tannerella forsythensis*, *Eikenella corrodens*, *P. gingivalis*, *P. intermedia and T. denticola* (Dahle et al. 1996; Sundqvist 1992; Rotstein and Simon 2004). *T. denticola, T. forsythia and P. gingivalis* can be found in endodontic infections and they are the 'red complex' of bacterial implicated in severe forms of periodontitis (Socransky and Haffajee 2005; Sundqvist 1994), therefore, subgingival plaque may be a source of root canal micro-organisms.

A recent systematic review of literature published within the last 10 years, reiterated that 'red' and 'orange' complex microbes were found in both root canals and periodontal pockets, suggesting that one site could be the source of infection for the other (Gambin et al. 2021). The presence of the red complex in endo-perio lesions was not found. The included data related to periodontal lesions with secondary endodontic involvement and true combined perio-endo lesions. The microbes most identified at both sites were *P. micra* (0.3–0.7 microns in size), *Eubacterium nodatum* (0.5–0.9 microns in size) and *Streptococcus constellatus* (0.5–1 micron in size), all from the 'orange' complex and small enough to enter dentinal tubules (1.7–4 microns in size) or via the apical foramen (240 microns in size). *P. micra*, a Gram-positive coccus, a strict anaerobe and a commensal, associated with chronic periodontitis and endocarditis, capable of inducing an intense inflammatory response (Gambin et al. 2021). *E. nodatum* is a Gram-positive, non-flagellated, non-sporulating rod, and is strictly anaerobic. *S. constellatus* (a Gram-positive encapsulated, non-flagellated coccus, a commensal, with anaerobic and microaerophilic metabolism) can colonise tissues such as the pulp and extraorally (where they are not usually found), can evade and survive the attack of neutrophils, degrade hyaluronate and chondroitin in connective tissue, as well as produce hydrogen sulphide which, not only helps resistance of pathogens to cell lysis but also immuno-modulatory actions (Gambin et al. 2021).

Our understanding of the oral microflora is ever evolving and new technologies are providing insight into their interactions, which may in time change our view of this complex relationship between the oral cavity and its inhabitants.

Before moving on to diagnosing periodontal and endodontic disease with manifestations of each other, the individual diseases must be understood.

References

Adriaens PA. Bacterial invasion in periodontitis, is it important in periodontal treatment? Rev Belg Med Dent. 1984;44:9–30.

Adriaens PA, Edwards CA, De Boever JA, Loesche WJ. Ultrastructural observations on bacterial invasion in cementum and radicular dentin of periodontally diseased human teeth. J Periodontol. 1988;59:493–503.

Armitage GC, Ryder MI, Wilcox SE. Cemental changes in teeth with heavily infected root canals. J Endod. 1983;9(4):127–30.

Athanassiadis B, Abbott PV, Walsh LJ. The use of calcium hydroxide, antibiotics and biocides as antimicrobial medicaments in endodontics. Aust Dent J Suppl. 2007;52(1 Suppl):S64–82.

Baugh D, Wallace J. The role of apical instrumentation in root canal treatment: a review of the literature. J Endod. 2005;31(5):333–40.

Carranza F, Newman M, Takei H. Carranza's clinical periodontology. 10th ed. St. Louis: Elsevier Saunders; 2006.

Cobb CM, Sottosanti JS. A re-evaluation of scaling and root planing. J Periodontol. 2021;92(10):1370–8.

Costerton JW, Stewart PS. Biofilms and device related infections. In: Nataro PJ, Basler MJ, Cunningham-Rundels S, editors. Persistent bacterial infections. Washington, DC: ASM Press; 2000. p. 423–39.

Curtis MA, Diaz PI, Van Dyke TE. The role of microbiota in periodontal disease. Perio. 2020;83:14–25.

Dahle UR, Tronstad L, Olsen I. Characterization of new periodontal and endodontic isolates of spirochetes. Eur J Oral Sci. 1996;104:41–7.

Donnermeyer D, Bürklein S, Dammaschke T, Schäfer E. Endodontic sealers based on calcium silicates: a systematic review. Odontology. 2019;107(4):421–36.

Feng Z, Weinberg A. Role of bacteria in health and disease of periodontal tissues. Periodontology. 2006;40:50–76.

Fine DH, Markowitz K, Furgang D, et al. Aggregatibacter actinomycetemcomitans and its relationship to initiation of localized aggressive periodontitis: longitudinal cohort study of initially healthy adolescents. J Clin Microbiol. 2007;45(12):3859–69.

Gambin DJ, Vitali FC, De Carli JP, Mazzon RR, Gomes BPFA, Duque TM, Trentin MS. Prevalence of red and orange microbial complexes in endodontic-periodontal lesions: a systematic review and meta-analysis. Clin Oral Investig. 2021;25(12):6533–46.

Haffajee AD, Socransky SS. Microbial etiological agents of destructive periodontal diseases. Periodontol. 1994;5:78–111.

Haffajee AD, Teles RP, Socransky SS. The effect of periodontal therapy on the composition of the subgingival microbiota. Periodontol 2000. 2006;42:219–58.

Haubek D, Ennibi OK, Poulsen K, Vaeth M, Poulsen S, Kilian M. Risk of aggressive periodontitis in adolescent carriers of the JP2 clone of Aggregatibacter (Actinobacillus) actinomycetemcomitans in Morocco: a prospective longitudinal cohort study. Lancet. 2008;371(9608):237–42.

Herrera D, Retamal-Valdes B, Alonso B, Feres M. Acute periodontal lesions (periodontal abscesses and necrotizing periodontal diseases) and endo-periodontal lesions. J Periodontol. 2018;89(Suppl 1):S85–S102.

Kakehashi S, Stanley HR, Fitzgerald RJ. The effects of surgical exposures of dental pulps in germ-free and conventional laboratory rats. Oral Surg Oral Med Oral Pathol. 1965;20:340–9.

Korzen BH, Krakow AA, Green DB. Pulpal and periapical tissue responses in conventional and mono- infected gnotobiotic rats. Oral Surg. 1974;37:783–802.

Mah TC, O'Toole GA. Mechanisms of biofilm resistance to antimicrobial agents. Trends Microbiol. 2001;9:34e9.

Moller AJ, Fabricius L, Dahlen G, Ohman AE, Heyden G. Influence on periapical tissues of indigenous oral bacteria and necrotic pulp tissue in monkeys. Scand J Dent Res. 1981;89:475–84.

Moore WE, Moore LV. The bacteria of periodontal diseases. Periodontology. 1994;5:66–77.

Nair PNR. Light and electron microscopic studies of root canal flora and periapical lesions. J Endod. 1987;13:29–39.

Paster BJ, Boches SK, Galvin JL, Ericson RE, Lau CN, Levanos VA, Sahasrabudhe A, Dewhirst FE. Bacterial diversity in Human Subgingival Plaque. J Bacteriol. 2001;183(12):3770–83.

Peeran SW, Thiruneervannan M, Abdalla KA, Mugrabi MH. Endo-perio lesions. Int J Sci Technol Res. 2013;2(5):268–74.

Portenier I, Waltimo TMT, Haapasalo M. *Enterococcus faecalis* – the root canal survivor and 'star' in post treatment disease. Endod Top. 2003;6:135–59.

Rotstein I, Simon JH. Diagnosis, prognosis and decision-making in the treatment of combined periodontal-endodontic lesions. Periodontol. 2004;34:165–203.

Rupf S, Kannengiesser S, Merte K, Pfister W, Sigusch B, Eschrich K. Comparison of profiles of key periodontal pathogens in periodontium and endodontium. Dent Traumatol. 2000;16(6):269–75.

Siqueira JF Jr, Rôças IN. Polymerase chain reaction-based analysis of microorganisms associated with failed endodontic treatment. Oral Surg Oral Med Oral Pathol Oral Radiol Endod. 2004;97(1):85–94.

Slots J, Taubman M. Contemporary oral microbiology and immunology. St. Louis: Mosby; 1992.

Socransky SS, Haffajee AD. Periodontal microbial ecology. Periodontol. 2005;38:135–87.

Socransky SS, Haffajee AD, Cugini MA, Smith C, Kent RL Jr. Microbial complexes in subgingival plaque. J Clin Periodontol. 1998;25(2):134–44.

Sundqvist G. Bacteriological studies of necrotic dental pulps. Umea: University of Umea; 1976. Dissertation

Sundqvist G. Associations between microbial species in dental root canal infections. Oral Microbiol Immunol. 1992;7:257–62.

Sundqvist G. Taxonomy, ecology, and pathogenicity of the root canal flora. Oral Surg Oral Med Oral Pathol. 1994;78:522–30.

Sundqvist G, Figdor D. Life as an endodontic pathogen. Endod Top. 2003;6(1):3–28.

Svensater G, Bergenholtz G. Biofilms in endodontic infections. Endod Top. 2004;9:27–36.

Torabinejad M, Ung B, Kettering JD. In vitro bacterial penetration of coronally unsealed endodontically treated teeth. J Endod. 1990;16:566–9.

Tronstad L, Sunde PT. The evolving new understanding of endodontic infections. Endod Top. 2003;6:55–77.

Van Winkelhoff AJ, van Steenbergen TJM, de Graaff J. The role of black-pigmented bacteroides in human oral infections. J Clin Periodontol. 1988;15(3):145–55.

Wilson M. Susceptibility of oral bacterial biofilms to antimicrobial agents. J Med Microbiol. 1996;44:79–87.

Zehnder M, Gold SI, Hasselgren G. Pathologic interaction in pulpal and periodontal tissues. J Clin Periodontol. 2002;29:663–71.

The Diagnosis, Management and Outcomes of Periodontal Lesions

4

Abstract

This chapter of the book briefly discusses periodontal disease, its management and the expected outcomes of treatment. This understanding can be extrapolated to the management of perio-endo lesions.

Periodontal Disease

Periodontitis can be considered a chronic inflammatory reaction to the presence of bacteria in genetically susceptible individuals, causing destruction of the periodontal attachment, usually commencing at the gingival sulcus and travelling apically (Cobb and Sottosanti 2021; Carranza et al. 2006; Genco 1992). Host responses to microbes and to treatment differ from individual to individual. Untreated periodontal disease will lead to the loss of the very foundations that maintain the teeth in the oral cavity and eventual loss of the affected teeth, which can have a significant impact on the psychosocial aspects and happiness of patients. When the quality of life of patients with periodontal disease was investigated, patients with periodontal disease had poorer perceived oral health (Needleman et al. 2004; Dannan and Joumaa 2015; Bhargava et al. 2021; Ferreira et al. 2017), and those with more than eight teeth with pockets deeper than 5 mm were said to have worse perceived oral health (Needleman et al. 2004; Cunha-cruz et al. 2007).

Periodontal disease affects 90% of the population to some degree. Longitudinal studies of between 100 and 600 patients, followed up for up to 53 years, show that approximately 80% of patients can be well maintained (with supportive periodontal care) and lose less than 3 teeth during the supportive periodontal care phase (Hirschfeld and Wasserman 1978; McFall 1982; Matuliene et al. 2008). Approximately ten percent of the population have been described as 'rapid/extreme

S. Eliyas, *The Periodontic-Endodontic Interface*,
https://doi.org/10.1007/978-3-031-49937-1_4

downhillers' (losing many teeth, despite all efforts). In these patients the disease is difficult to manage. Equally, these patients are difficult to identify early, therefore, the benefit of the doubt should be given (Hirschfeld and Wasserman 1978; McFall 1982; Loe et al. 1986).

During early periodontitis, the junctional epithelium will migrate apically along the root surface and form a periodontal pocket. The collagen in the periodontal ligament has a very high rate of turnover, and therefore, any inflammation can cause rapid loss of the supporting tissue of the tooth (Nanci 2008). Periodontal treatment is not curative and is aimed at helping the patient to manage the condition and prevent further destruction. Often the periodontal treatment does not restore the entire periodontal architecture, with formation of a long junctional epithelium at best, and pocket reduction occurring through a combination of regeneration and recession, the latter being more probable. These patients are likely to be lifelong patients. There is a large role for the profession to play in patient motivation and giving the patient ownership of their disease. It is the patient's oral hygiene that is likely to make the largest impact on disease progression. Other factors that affect the outcome include genetic susceptibility, smoking, stress, systemic disease, age, gender, furcation involvements, baseline bone loss and use of the tooth as an abutment (Eickholz et al. 2008; Pretzl et al. 2008). Local factors that trap plaque, such as overhangs, can also cause localised periodontal destruction in those not necessarily prone to periodontal disease.

The Diagnosis of Periodontal Disease

History taking in periodontal patients may reveal the presence of bleeding on brushing, recession, movement and splaying of teeth, but often not pain, unless there is an acute exacerbation (Fig. 4.1a, b). The diagnosis of periodontal disease includes the clinical and radiographic assessment of the periodontal tissues. The following assessments should be made to identify the presence of periodontitis and understand the possible aetiology.

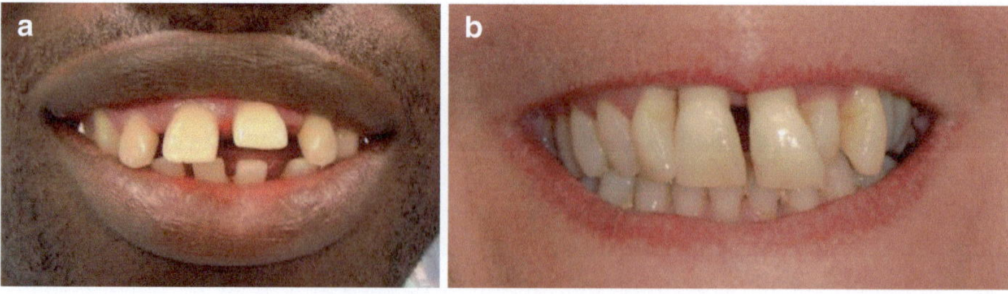

Fig. 4.1 Extra-oral photographs showing that presentations of periodontal disease can be challenging to manage. (**a**) Splayed teeth and (**b**) long teeth, especially in those with a high lip line

Plaque and Gingival Scores

The visual presence or absence of plaque (plaque scores) is often used to judge the patient's ability to maintain good oral hygiene. The presence of plaque on occlusal surfaces of teeth is less relevant to periodontal disease than plaque at the gingival margin. The Plaque Index recommends that the thickness of the plaque at the gingival margin be scored 0–3 (Silness and Loe 1964). It must be noted that plaque scores are a snap shot in time, because a patient may have a low plaque score if he/she brushed well on the day of the appointment, although, this does not mean the patient brushes well on the other days when a plaque score is not being measured. The better index may be the Gingival Index, which scores the amount of gingival inflammation and bleeding, and the absence of inflammation in most cases is more reflective of continued good oral hygiene (Loe and Silness 1963).

Bleeding and Suppuration

Bleeding on probing as a measure may give some idea about the presence of inflammation. It must be noted that smokers may not necessarily show frank bleeding on probing despite the presence of plaque and deep periodontal pockets. Average bleeding on probing at 25% of sites has been considered the highest acceptable value for adequately maintaining healthy gingival conditions (Lang et al. 1986). Bleeding on probing is not an indicator for disease progression (Badersten et al. 1985; Lang et al. 1986), but the absence of bleeding on probing can be seen as a good criterion for the maintenance of periodontal stability (Lang et al. 1990). It has been stated that at the end of supportive periodontal therapy, the percentage of the total sites with bleeding on probing can be as low as 2.1% (Carnevale et al. 2007) and that it was possible to achieve a mean reduction in bleeding on probing of approximately 45% for 4–6.5 mm pockets following mechanical non-surgical periodontal treatment (Cobb 2002).

Suppuration from a pocket will indicate the presence of infection as well as inflammation. Suppuration does not necessarily indicate infection related only to periodontal disease. Endodontic infections can also present with suppuration at the gingival crevice, and this is discussed later in the book.

Periodontal Pocket Depths

Periodontal pocket depths are measured to gain an understanding of the depth of the pocket as it not only indicates the presence of periodontal breakdown, but also the likelihood of improvement with oral hygiene measures and active periodontal therapy. It has been suggested that there might be a difference in 'clinical' measurement of the pocket depth and that seen 'histologically', with the extent of tissue penetration being affected by the thickness of the probe, the pressure applied, contour of the tooth surface, the degree of inflammatory cell infiltrate and accompanying loss of collagen fibres, as well as the presence of tears in the junctional epithelium (Listgarten 1980).

The 'walking' of a 0.5 mm diameter ball ended probe with a force of 20 g or 0.25 N around individual teeth to identify periodontal pockets has been recommended as not to traumatise the tissues. The performance of a Basic Periodontal Examination (BPE) is recommended for all patients at regular intervals (Ainamo et al. 1982; British Society of Periodontology 2011; 2019; Chapple et al. 2018). A number of different periodontal probes have been recommended, with the World Health Organisation (WHO), Williams and Florida probes (Florida Probe Corp, Gainesville, FL) being the most popular. The Florida Probe may have better accuracy (Hefti 1997; Al Shayeb et al. 2014; Gupta et al. 2015).

In health, the periodontal probe is likely to stop short of reaching the most coronal connective tissue fibres of the pocket or sulcus, which should start 0.4 mm coronal to the junctional epithelium. In gingivitis, the probe stays 0.1 mm coronal to the junctional epithelium, and in periodontitis the probe penetrates between 0.25 and 0.5 mm past the apical termination of the junctional epithelium (Listgarten 1980). Therefore, periodontal pocket measurement can be an inaccurate measurement of the anatomical sulcus/pocket with an estimated error of 1–2 mm, and the error could be up to the entire length of long junctional epithelium formed following treatment (Listgarten 1980; Badersten et al. 1984a; Armitage 1999). In disease the junctional epithelium may be more permeable, therefore, giving an over estimate of the pocket probing depth, and following periodontal treatment, resolution of inflammation at the gingival margin may lead to an underestimate of the true pocket depth (Badersten et al. 1984a). Therefore, finding single deep pockets in diagnosing period-endo lesions may be more difficult in those patients who have undergone periodontal treatment and achieved stability.

Periodontal pockets of 0–3 mm are considered healthy, and pockets >4 mm may pose difficulties for patients to clean. It has been shown that residual pockets of 4 mm or deeper bleed more frequently than sites with probing depths of less than 4 mm (Lang et al. 1986), reflecting these difficulties. Residual pockets of 6 mm and numerous pockets of 5 mm with bleeding on probing are considered a risk for the progression of periodontal disease (Matuliene et al. 2008).

Recession and Clinical Attachment Level

The lack of periodontal pocketing is not reassurance that the patient is not susceptible to periodontal disease. The important measurement is clinical attachment level. This requires the measurement of recession and periodontal pocket depth, the addition of both give the clinical attachment loss. Following periodontal treatment, the reduction in pocket depth is attributed to a combination of gain in clinical attachment level and gingival recession. Recession is measured from the cemento-enamel junction to the gingival margin. In a patient without generalised periodontal pockets, a single pocket may suggest endodontic involvement, however, the presence of generalised recession may signify a susceptibility to periodontal disease, which is now generally stable. Recession defects can be classified using a variety of indices depending on the height and width of the defect, involvement of the mucogingival junction and the presence of interproximal attachment loss (Miller Jr. 1985; Cairo et al. 2011).

Mobility

The most commonly used classification for mobility of teeth is using a scale of 0–3 (Miller 1950). Zero is physiological mobility (0.1–0.2 mm in a horizontal direction), the absence of which may indicate replacement resorption and/or ankylosis. Ankylosed teeth usually sound different, with a metallic or high-pithed sound (Lin et al. 2022). A score of 1 denotes less than 1 mm horizontal movement, 2 denotes more than 1 mm horizontal movement and 3 denotes the presence of both horizontal and vertical movement. The presence of mobility may not necessarily be related to periodontal attachment loss from marginal gingival breakdown, but could also be related to periodontal attachment loss from apical or periradicular inflammation/infection or as a result of occlusal trauma/fremitus. Residual mobility after periodontal treatment has been shown not to lead to further bone loss (Hirschfeld and Wasserman 1978; Polson 1980); it may be the inconvenience to the patient that leads to removal of the tooth.

Furcation Involvements

There are a number of classifications that have been used to express the presence, extent and characteristics of a furcation involvement (Pilloni and Rojas 2018). The presence of a furcation involvement might suggest difficulty in oral hygiene due to root morphology, but could equally imply the presence of endodontic infections communicating via perforations, furcal or lateral canals. The extent and characteristics of a furcation will determine the ability to treat, manage or regenerate the defect. The presence of furcations have always been used to determine prognosis, however, the dental profession has not necessarily been seen to accurately predict tooth loss in periodontal patients (McFall 1982; Hirschfeld and Wasserman 1978; Nibali et al. 2016).

Hirschfeld and Wasserman (1978) reported that 17% of teeth with 'questionable' prognosis were lost in the 'Well Maintained' group, whereas, in the 'Extreme Downhillers' group almost all of teeth with 'questionable' prognosis were lost. Interestingly, 20% of all teeth lost in all of the groups combined, included teeth that were not deemed 'questionable', and were those that were maintained for many years and suddenly developed periodontal destruction. McFall reported (1982) that teeth deemed of 'questionable' prognosis were lost during maintenance with about 27% of teeth in the 'Well Maintained' group and 91.8% in 'Extreme Downhillers' group being lost during this time. 56% of teeth with a favourable prognosis were lost, 57% of questionable teeth with furcations were lost (therefore 43% were not) and 64% of questionable teeth without furcations were also lost. Think about the root morphology and cleansability of the furcation when considering prognosis.

Radiographic Examination

With the new classification of periodontal disease, radiographic examination has taken a more prominent role (European Federation of Periodontology 2019). Previously, radiographs were useful in understanding the level of bone destruction, and sometimes the progression of periodontal disease if sequential radiographs from different time points were available for the same patient. Although dental panoramic tomography is often used as a screening tool, long cone periapical radiographs of teeth with deep periodontal pockets are necessary for accurate treatment planning. Plain film radiographs can underestimate the depth and pattern of the defect, and cone beam computed tomography (CBCT) offers a more accurate understanding of the defect, as well as enabling the visualization of apical lesions, resorption and perio-endo lesions (Walter and Sculean 2016). However, the slightly increased dose must be justified with its impact on decision-making: will the CBCT add to the clinical and plain film radiographic findings, and therefore, alter the treatment plan? In time, reduction in dose and improvement in technology may mean CBCTs become the primary mode of radiographic assessment.

Bone Sounding

With local anaesthesia, it is also possible to probe the tissues, until the probe encounters bone. This is advised in inflamed periodontal pockets that are due to have surgical treatment, especially to better appreciate the nature of bony defect. This helps to mentally visualise the defect and remaining walls, which may alter the treatment plan and help decide between treatments such as regenerative periodontal surgery and pocket reduction periodontal surgery. Bone sounding is not recommended after treatment, as this may damage the healing periodontal pocket.

The Management of Periodontal Disease

The management of periodontal disease may span from patient motivation and education, professional debridement of pockets to supportive periodontal care. Monitoring and understanding the progression of the disease is a paramount part of the management (Case 10).

Case 10 A 56-year-old male patient presented with vertical bone defects associated with teeth that 6 years previously showed good bone levels. The disease appears to have developed and progressed significantly over a relatively short period of time. Bitewing radiographs from 2000 (Fig. 4.2a, b) and 2003 (Fig. 4.3a, b) reveal relatively small/early vertical defects associated with the first permanent molars. The bone loss progresses rapidly from 2006 (Fig. 4.4) to 2009 (Fig. 4.5) with little change in the restoration present in the lower first molars, the restoration in the upper left first molar has been renewed and is larger, and the bone levels associated with the distal aspect of the lower left second molar cannot be seen on the bitewing radiographs.

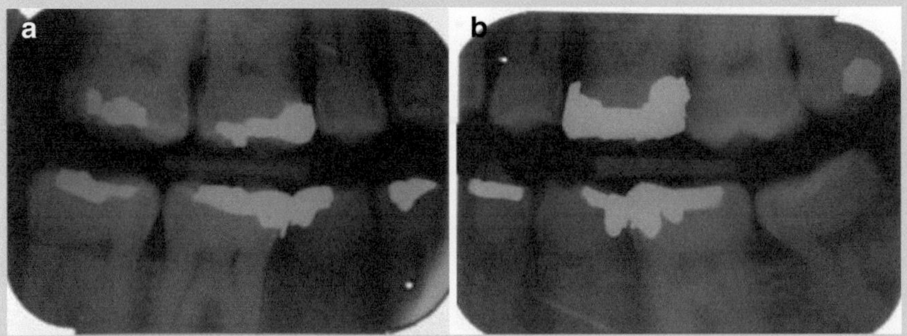

Fig. 4.2 Right (**a**) and left (**b**) bitewing radiographs showing good bone levels around molar teeth in 2000

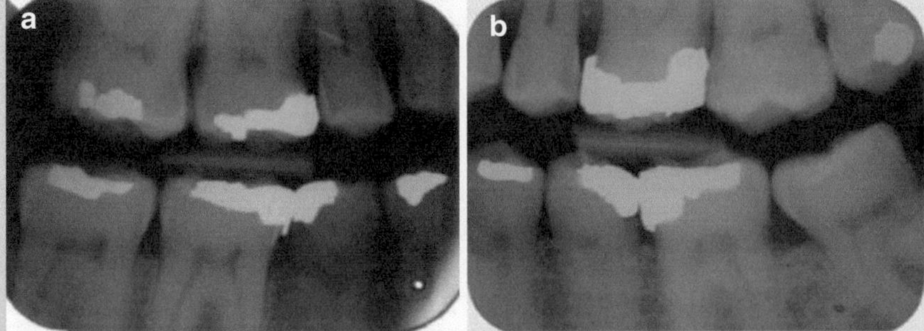

Fig. 4.3 Right (**a**) and left (**b**) bitewing radiographs showing early signs of vertical bone defects associated with the mesial aspect of the LR6 and distal aspect of the LL6 in 2003, although in these areas the restorations have not changed

Fig. 4.4 Left bitewing radiograph showing progression of the vertical defect on the distal aspect of the LL6 in 2006

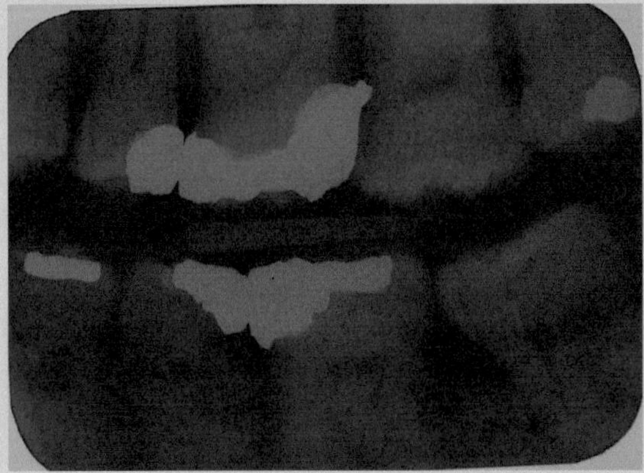

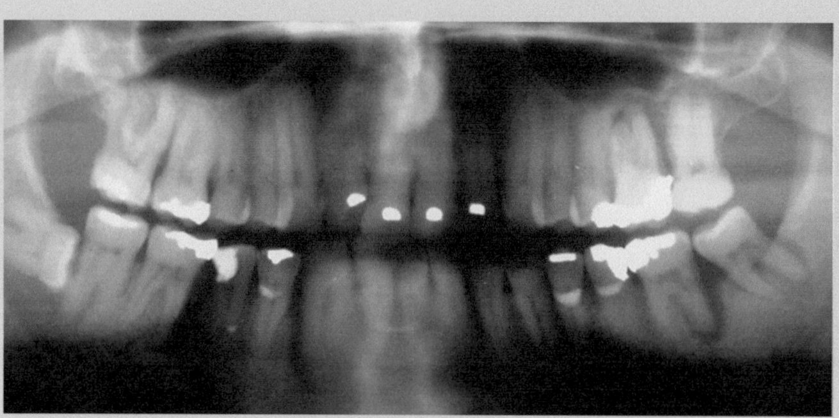

Fig. 4.5 DPT showing significant progression of the vertical defects associated with the mesial aspect of the LR6, distal aspects of the LL6, UL6 and UR6

Active Treatment

The most vital part of the management of periodontal disease involves oral health education (especially with regard to oral hygiene instructions, diabetic control and smoking cessation), removal of local plaque retentive factors and disturbance of the plaque biofilm/reduction of the critical mass of plaque bacteria (Cobb 2002). Treatment may include non-surgical and surgical root surface debridement (RSD) with or without adjunctive antibiotics, surgical regeneration or alteration of root morphology via root amputation/root resection.

Non-surgical periodontal treatment is now regarded as root surface debridement and not root planing, with ultrasonic instruments for speed and possibly full mouth debridement within 24 hours (Quirynen et al. 2006). Patient factors (such as inability to tolerate long appointment and anxiety) and treatment factors (such as the need for adjunctive antibiotics) may influence the way active periodontal treatment is delivered. Although, it may seem sensible to delay providing active treatment until oral hygiene is optimal, the presence of plaque retentive factors can hinder oral hygiene. Sometimes the use of 24 hours debridement will not only reduce the microbial load in one sitting, but also serve as a strong motivating factor in improving patient compliance. In those with heart disease it may be appropriate to provide quadrant-wise debridement, as consideration has been given recently to increased levels of C-Reactive Proteins present after root surface debridement (Sanz et al. 2020).

In relation to the various aspects of periodontal treatment, reviews by Cobb (2002) and Cobb and Sottosanti (2021) made the following observations:

- The correct use of hand scalers may achieve the same result as ultrasonic/sonic instruments, however, the latter has been shown to be 20–50% faster at reaching the same clinical end point. Sonic and ultrasonic scalers can generate more aerosols and tactile sensation can be reduced. No difference in pocket depth improvement, bleeding on probing, clinical attachment level with the use of hand/sonic/ ultrasonic instruments has been shown by some (Wenstrom et al. 2005). However, the use of hand instruments is time consuming and technique sensitive, with need for correct and frequent instrument sharpening. Some studies have demonstrated difficulties cleaning pockets that are deeper than 5 mm with either instrument, and that reaching the apex of these pockets were rare, however, other studies have shown that ultrasonic and 'microultrasonic' instruments have the ability to clean the apical extent of pockets that are 4–6 mm deep and those that are 7 mm or deeper as well as clean furcations better (Beuchat et al. 2001). Scaling efficacy reduces with increase in pocket depth, presence of concavities, grooves, restoration contours and extent of furcations. It is reported that sonic and ultrasonic instruments produce less tooth surface loss (Ritz et al. 1991). Deeper pockets may benefit from open flap debridement early on in the active treatment phase rather than a second (or even first) cycle of non-surgical periodontal treatment (Fardal et al. 2004; Checchi et al. 2002; Heitz-Mayfield et al. 2002). It is not often possible to remove all bacterial plaque and calculus from a pocket, and with current instrumentation, it is not possible to achieve root surface smoothness required to prevent bacterial colonization. Plaque control alone is thought to produce no or minimal reduction in clinical inflammation without active periodontal treatment. There is also a thought that prolonged scaling may introduce bacteria into areas not yet infected.

- The presence of bacteria in cementum and root dentine, and the presence of certain groups of bacteria (*A. actinomycetemcomitans*, *P. gingivalis* and *T. denticola*) may preclude pocket healing because of their ability to invade the periodontal tissues. Complete removal of infected cementum is considered unrealistic and unnecessary. Subgingival scaling has been shown to reduce Gram negative bacteria and allow thriving of Gram positive rods and cocci required for health, however, the shift in bacteria towards health may be transient and regular debridement is required during supportive periodontal care.

- Studies have shown that debridement carried out over numerous visits, weeks apart or within 24 hours has little impact on long-term outcome. Other studies have shown that 24 hours full mouth disinfection (with full mouth scaling and root planing in less than 24 hours, pocket irrigation with 1% chlorhexidine gel 3 times in 10 minutes, oral rinsing with 0.2% chlorhexidine twice a day for 1 minutes for 14 days and daily tongue brushing) reduced probing depths by 1.4 mm in multi-rooted teeth and 2.3 mm in single rooted teeth. This change was maintained at 8 months post treatment. Although, more recent studies have shown no difference (Eberhard et al. 2008).

- The largest changes in pocket depths occurs in the first 1–3 months, with healing and maturation of the gingival tissues continuing for 9–12 months. Measurements taken prematurely may lead to conclusions that treatment has been unsuccessful; when in reality more time is required for healing. This may pose a dilemma when periodontal treatment is required for perio-endo lesions, with signs of infection and the opportunity at multiple endodontic treatment visits to provide root surface debridement. Provision of root surface debridement repeatedly, at each endodontic appointment, may be counter-productive as healing may continually be disrupted.

Current thinking is around effective personalised oral health education (including smoking cessation advice, referral for diabetic control and oral hygiene instructions), root surface debridement of pockets 4 mm or deeper under local anaesthesia (depending on the number of sites, the non-surgical root surface debridement can take several hours to complete as 2 minutes of debridement per site has been suggested) and re-assessment at 3 months after active treatment (Cobb and Sottosanti 2021). Care should be taken when ultrasonic scalers are used for this length of time (Fig. 7.2). New guidance recommends Professional Mechanical Plaque Removal (PMPR) and indicates a place for supragingival scaling, subgingival scaling (both of which identifies and removal plaque retentive factors and calculus) and debridement, which systematically washes and cleans endotoxin related cementum (West et al. 2021). In this new guidance, treatment is recommended in steps, depending on patient compliance and motivation.

Oral hygiene is the cornerstone of managing periodontal disease (Fig. 4.6). Patients skilled with the use of interdental brushes and single tufted brushes may be able to reach the base of a 5 mm periodontal pocket, but not deeper. The importance of the daily disturbance of the biofilm of bacteria using single tufted brushes (Fig. 4.6a) and 'snug-fitting' interdental brushes (Fig. 4.6b–d) placed at the gingival margin cannot be stressed enough. As healing occurs, recession of the gingival tissues is likely. The interdental brushes must follow this new gingival position to be effective.

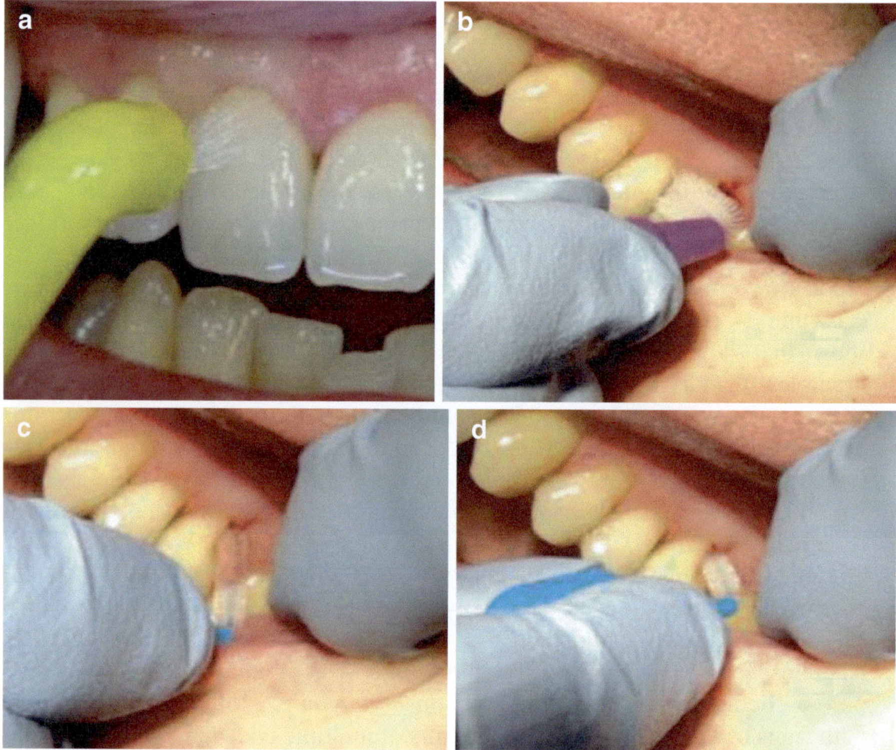

Fig. 4.6 Intra-oral photographs showing the use of single tufted brush (**a**), interdental brushes at gingival level (**b**), interdental brushes in furcation areas (**c** and **d**)

After the first cycle of root surface debridement, the majority of the change in pocket size is likely to be as a result of resolution of inflammation with a small element of attachment gain. As evidence suggests that deep pockets are not debrided well, even with focused water spray and the use of slim ultrasonic tips (Caffesse et al. 1986; Rabbani et al. 1981), one cycle of root surface debridement may reduce the depth of deep pockets, so that the base of these pockets may be more accessible during the second cycle of root surface debridement. A second cycle may allow removal of missed calculus, although, it is appreciated that the first cycle gives the best opportunity for access into the pocket due to the gingival tissues being inflamed and loose. After the first cycle it is likely that these gingival tissues will form a tight cuff around the tooth as the inflammation resolves and healing begins (Badersten et al. 1984b). There is evidence to show that a second cycle of root surface debridement does not necessarily always give further improvement (Badersten et al. 1984b; Anderson et al. 1996). In a poorly motivated patient, it may not be ideal to provide surgical treatment and a second cycle of root surface debridement may be more appropriate. In a well-motivated patient with excellent oral hygiene, the need for surgical periodontal treatment after the first cycle of root surface debridement should be considered (Fardal et al. 2004; Checchi et al. 2002). In some cases of deep pockets, it may be appropriate to consider surgical periodontal treatment from the start, as it is not expected that the base such deep pockets will be reached by any of the instruments during non-surgical root surface debridement.

Surgical Periodontal Treatment

Surgical periodontal treatment may be in the way of access to deep pockets with open flap debridement leading to pocket reduction and healing, with recession and some level of clinical attachment gain (Carranza et al. 2006). Surgical periodontal treatment may also be resective, where a width of gingival tissue is removed, thereby artificially reducing the depth of the pocket, although there may also be healing with clinical attachment gain, as debridement of the pocket with direct visual access will have been completed as part of the procedure (Carranza et al. 2006). Surgical periodontal treatment may also be regenerative, where there is a combination of open flap debridement and placement of regenerative materials within the infrabony defect to facilitate regeneration of the periodontal tissues (Needleman et al. 2006). No significant difference in longterm outcomes of non-surgical and surgical periodontal treatment have been reported by some (Pihlstrom et al. 1983; Ramfjord et al. 1987a, b; Antczak-Bouckoms et al. 1993), and others have shown better reduction in pockets depths with surgical treatment for those periodontal pockets that are deeper than 7 mm (Heitz-Mayfield et al. 2002). Regenerative treatment can result in long-term retention of teeth with infrabony defects and associated deep pockets (Cortellini and Tonetti 2004; Pretzl et al. 2008; Nygaard-Østby et al. 2010).

It must be remembered that scaling and root planing will expose dentinal tubules to some extent, and the bacteria usually remain within the outermost third of the root dentine (Adriaens et al. 1988), and they are unlikely to cause significant pulpal irritation due to the host defence system within a healthy pulp, however these reservoirs of bacteria may re-enter a cleaned periodontal pocket (Chapple and Lumley 1999).

Adjunctive Antibiotics

Antibiotics have been shown to be useful in pocket depth reduction for periodontal disease as an adjunct to scaling and root planing (Haffajee et al. 2003, 2007; Guerrero et al. 2005; Griffiths et al. 2011; Oteo et al. 2010), with it being more cost effective when used systemically (Heasman et al. 2011). A systematic review on the use of adjunctive antibiotics when providing root surface debridement showed that antibiotics only offer additional benefit when used in patients with deep pockets, active sites, aggressive disease and with specific microbiological profiles (Herrera et al. 2002; Herrera et al. 2008). Often used antibiotics are doxycycline, metronidazole, amoxicillin and azithromycin, although there are many (Haas et al. 2008; Kapoor et al. 2012). The absorption with oral intake can be varied, from 90% with metronidazole, 75% with amoxicillin and 37% with azithromycin (Soares et al. 2015; Foulds et al. 1996; Turgut and Özyazici 2004). Azithromycin needs to be taken 1 hours before or 2 hours after food as this affects bioavailability (Foulds et al. 1996). Antibiotics such as metronidazole and amoxycillin are usually prescribed for 7–14 days and expected to be administered three time a day, where as azithromycin can be taken once a day for three days starting on the day of treatment. They can also be used as topical applications into the periodontal pocket (doxycycline and metronidazole). The reactions and resistance to antibiotics should be considered prior to their use. Antibiotics are usually not recommended as part of routine endodontic treatment (Cope et al. 2018), and therefore, would not generally be recommended as part of the treatment of perio-endo lesions, unless the periodontal disease component of the lesion calls for their use.

Supportive Periodontal Therapy

Supportive periodontal therapy is usually considered recurring re-assessment, oral health education as well as supra and subgingival PMPR as required (often at 3 or 4 monthly intervals depending on the patient's needs). Patients that were erratically compliant with maintenance programmes were said to have a 5.6 fold increase in risk of tooth loss than those who were regularly compliant (Checchi et al. 2002). Eickholz et al. (2008) and Pretzl et al. (2008) showed that without supportive periodontal therapy, the number of teeth lost was increased. Some have shown no difference in pocket depth reduction or clinical attachment levels when using supragingival or subgingival scaling during the supportive periodontal care phase (Heasman et al. 2002). Supportive periodontal therapy in longitudinal studies has not only included oral health education and root surface debridement of pockets that are 4 mm or deeper, but also, surgical periodontal treatment and root amputation/resection when required (Hirschfeld and Wasserman 1978; McFall 1982). Teeth with even severe periodontal disease can be retained with strict supportive periodontal care (Lindhe and Nyman 1984; Pretzl et al. 2008; Huynh-Ba et al. 2009; Chambrone et al. 2010; Leininger et al. 2010; Bäumer et al. 2011; Ng et al. 2011). The retention of 'hopeless' teeth do not seem to negatively impact the remaining dentition in a well maintained patient (DeVore et al. 1988; Machtei et al. 1992; Wojcik et al. 1992; Machtei and Hirsch 2007).

The Outcome of Periodontal Treatment/Management

The outcome of periodontal treatment may be dependent on a variety of aspects including patient related factors such as susceptibility, age, smoking, stress, systemic disease, oral hygiene and treatment related factors (Eickholz et al. 2008; Pretzl et al. 2008). Treatment related factors include what information is given to patients regarding smoking cessation and oral hygiene, type of treatment provided such as non-surgical and surgical root surface debridement (with or without adjunctive antibiotics) and surgical regeneration. The outcome of periodontal treatment is measured via surrogate and true end points, as well as patient related outcomes. Surrogate end points measured are usually the number of bleeding sites present and the reduction of periodontal pockets depths, in terms of number of deep sites and the reduction of individual periodontal pocket depths. The expected change in pocket depths with active periodontal treatment is shown in Table 4.1. As can be seen, root surface debridement of shallow periodontal pockets can lead to loss of clinical attachment.

The true end point of periodontal disease and endodontic disease is tooth loss (Hujoel and DeRouen 1995), however, it is of advantage to ensure that teeth remain healthy within the oral cavity, rather than just being retained regardless of the state of infection. Studies have shown that periodontal disease is related to systemic health (Cullinan and Seymour 2009) and negatively impacts quality of life (Ferreira et al. 2017). The rate of tooth loss depends on the treatment philosophy: when large numbers of unpredictable teeth are extracted during active periodontal therapy phase, it is likely that a smaller number of teeth will be extracted during supportive periodontal therapy phase (Konig et al. 2002; McGuire 1991). It has been recommended that periodontal treatment should be evaluated based on overall tooth mortality and not only periodontal tooth mortality. This is because there is uncertainty as to whether the treatment itself influences mortality as a result of other causes, for example a tooth may fail due to development of caries in root dentine, which was only exposed to the oral environment as a result of surgery to make a furcation defect more cleansable (Hujoel et al. 1999).

Studies have suggested a correlation between individual tooth prognosis and rates of tooth loss for periodontal disease (Checchi et al. 2002). Teeth are usually considered of 'good', 'guarded/questionable/uncertain' or 'poor' prognosis. This is a subjective clinical judgment likely to be influenced by the experience and skill of the practitioner. Some say predicting which teeth should be extracted during

Table 4.1 Generally the expected pocket depth reduction with mechanical instrumentation is larger in deeper pockets (Cobb 1996)

Pocket depth at start of treatment	Mean reduction in pocket depth	Mean change in attachment level	Attachment after treatment
1-3mm pockets	0.03mm	- 0.34mm	Lost
4-6mm pockets	1.29mm	+ 0.55mm	Gained
7mm + pockets	2.16mm	+ 1.19mm	Gained

periodontal therapy is more accurate where teeth with good prognosis are involved (McGuire and Nunn 1999); others say that hopeless prognosis is more accurate in predicting tooth loss (McLeod et al. 1998). It has been shown that although the majority of teeth lost due to periodontal reasons in the supportive therapy period had an initial prognosis of uncertain, poor or hopeless, there were some teeth lost that initially deemed of good prognosis (Fardal et al. 2004; Checchi et al. 2002). Table 4.2 summarises some of the literature that has evaluated tooth loss during active periodontal treatment and that during supportive periodontal care.

Table 4.2 The percentage of teeth patients lost during different stages of treatment

Study	Review period	Inclusions/ exclusions	% tooth loss during active Tx	% tooth loss during SPT	% Overall tooth loss
Hirschfeld & Wasserman (1978)	15-53 years			8.4%	
McFall (1982)	15-29 years			11.4%	
Lindhe and Nyman (1984)	14 years				2.3%
Goldman et al. (1986)	15-34 years			13.4%	
Wood et al. (1989)	10-34 years			7.2%	
McLeod et al. (1997)	5-29 years			7.6%	
Kocher et al. (2000)	7 years	Periodontally untreated patients	3.4%	13.2%	16.6%
		Non-compliant patients	2.1%	12.5%	14.5%
		Compliant patients	4.3%	4%	8.3%
		Total patients in study	3.3%	9.1%	12.4%
Tonetti et al. (2000)	5.6 years	Including third molars & retained primary teeth	4.8%	4%	8.8%
Koing et al. (2002)	11.7 years	Excluded third molars & retained primary teeth	5%	2.9%	7.9%
Checchi et al. (2002)	3-12 years	Third molars were excluded	5.45%	2.16%	7.61%
Fardal et al. (2004)	9-11 years			1.5%	
Carnevale et al. 2007	3-17 years			0.9%	7.5%
Eickholz et al. 2008	10 years		2.4%	6.7%	9.1%

It is difficult to generalise the success of periodontal treatment due to the inherent measurement errors, surrogate end points, patient compliance, and difficulty in predicting the prognosis which influence treatment and extraction protocols. However, the majority of patients appear not to lose a large number of teeth, and therefore, it is worthwhile investing time and resources in providing active periodontal treatment and supportive periodontal care.

References

Adriaens PA, De Boever JA, Loesche WJ. Bacterial invasion in root cementum and radicular dentin of periodontally diseased teeth in humans. A reservoir of periodontopathic bacteria. J Periodontol. 1988;59:222–30.

Ainamo J, Barmes D, Beagrie G, Cutress T, Martin J, Sardo-Infirri J. Development of the World Health Organization (WHO) community periodontal index of treatment needs (CPITN). Int Dent J. 1982;32:281–91.

Al Shayeb KN, Turner W, Gillam DG. Accuracy and reproducibility of probe forces during simulated periodontal pocket depth measurements. Saudi Dent J. 2014;26(2):50–5.

Anderson GB, Palmer JA, Bye FL, Smith BA, Caffesse RG. Effectiveness of subgingival scaling and root planing: Single versus multiple episodes of instrumentation. J Periodontol. 1996;67:367–73.

Antczak-Bouckoms A, Joshipura K, Burdick E, Tulloch JF. Meta-analysis of surgical versus nonsurgical methods of treatment for periodontal disease. J Clin Periodontol. 1993;20(4):259–68.

Armitage GC. Development of a classification system for periodontal diseases and conditions. Ann Periodontol. 1999;4:1–6.

Badersten A, Nilvéaus R, Egelberg J. Reproducibility of probing attachment level measurements. J Clin Periodontol. 1984a;11(7):475–85.

Badersten A, Nilveus R, Egelberg J. Effect of nonsurgical periodontal therapy. III. Single versus repeated scaling and root planing. J Clin Periodontol. 1984b;11:114–24.

Badersten A, Nilveus R, Egelberg J. Effect of non-surgical periodontal therapy VII. Bleeding, suppuration and probing depths in sites with probing attachment loss. J Clin Periodontol. 1985;12:432–40.

Bäumer A, El Sayed N, Kim TS, Reitmeir P, Eickholz P, Pretzl B. Patient-related risk factors for tooth loss in aggressive periodontitis after active periodontal therapy. J Clin Periodontol. 2011;38:347–54.

Beuchat M, Busslinger A, Schmidlin PR, Michel B, Lehmann B, Lutz F. Clinical comparison of the effectiveness of novel sonic instruments and curettes for periodontal debridement after 2 months. J Clin Periodontol. 2001;28(12):1145–50.

Bhargava N, Jadhav A, Kumar P, Kapoor A, Mudrakola DP, Singh S. Oral health-related quality of life and severity of periodontal. Disease J Pharm Bioallied Sci. 2021;13(Suppl 1):S387–90.

British Society of Periodontology (BSP). Basic Periodontal Examination (BPE). London: BSP; 2011. https://www.bsperio.org.uk/assets/downloads/BPE_Guidelines_2011.pdf. Last accessed 22 July 2023]

British Society of Periodontology (BSP). Basic Periodontal Examination (BPE). London: BSP; 2019. https://www.bsperio.org.uk/assets/downloads/BSP_BPE_Guidelines_2019.pdf. Last accessed 22 July 2023]

Caffesse RG, Sweeney PL, Smith BA. Scaling and root planing with and without periodontal flap surgery. J Clin Periodontol. 1986;13(3):205–10.

Cairo F, Nieri M, Cincinelli S, Mervelt J, Pagliaro U. The interproximal clinical attachment level to classify gingival recessions and predict root coverage outcomes: an explorative and reliability study. J Clin Periodontol. 2011;38(7):661–6.

Carnevale G, Cairo F, Tonetti MS. Long term effects of supportive therapy in periodontal patients treated with fibre retention osseous resective surgery. 1: recurrence of pockets, bleeding on probing and tooth loss. J Clin Periodontology. 2007;34:334–41.

Carranza F, Newman M, Takei H. Carranza's clinical periodontology. 10th ed. St. Louis: Elsevier Saunders; 2006.

Chambrone L, Chambrone D, Lima LA, Chambrone LA. Predictors of tooth loss during long-term periodontal maintenance: a systematic review of observational studies. J Clin Periodontol. 2010;37(7):675–84.

Chapple ILC, Lumley PJ. The perio-endo interface. Dent Update. 1999;26:331–41.

Chapple ILC, Mealey BL, Van Dyke TE, et al. Periodontal health and gingival diseases and conditions on an intact and a reduced periodontium: consensus report of workgroup 1 of the 2017 World workshop on the classification of periodontal and peri-implant diseases and conditions. J Periodontol. 2018;89(Suppl 1):S74–84.

Checchi L, Montevecchi M, Gatto MR, Trombelli L. Retrospective study of tooth loss in 92 treated periodontal patients. J Clin Periodontol. 2002;29(7):651–6.

Cobb CM. Non-surgical pocket therapy: mechanical. Ann Periodontol. 1996;1(1):443–90.

Cobb CM. Clinical significance of non-surgical periodontal therapy: an evidence based perspective of scaling and root planing. J Clin Periodontol. 2002;29(S2):6–16.

Cobb CM, Sottosanti JS. A re-evaluation of scaling and root planing. J Periodontol. 2021;92(10):1370–8.

Cope AL, Francis N, Wood F, Chestnutt IG. Systemic antibiotics for symptomatic apical periodontitis and acute apical abscess in adults. Cochrane Database Syst Rev. 2018;9(9):CD010136.

Cortellini P, Tonetti MS. Long-term tooth survival following regenerative treatment of intrabony defects. J Periodontol. 2004;75(5):672–8.

Cullinan MP, Seymour GJ. Periodontal disease and systemic health: current status. Aust Dent J. 2009;54(1 Suppl):S62–9.

Cunha-Cruz J, Hujoel PP, Kressin NR. Oral health-related quality of life of periodontal patients. J Periodontal Res. 2007;42:169–76.

Dannan A, Joumaa A. Oral Health – related quality of life of periodontal patients in a Syrian sample – a pilot study. J Dent Oral Care Med. 2015;1(1):103.

DeVore CH, Beck FM, Horton JE. Retained "hopeless" teeth. Effects on the proximal periodontium of adjacent teeth. J Periodontol. 1988;59(10):647–51.

Eberhard J, Jervøe-Storm PM, Needleman I, Worthington H, Jepsen S. Full-mouth treatment concepts for chronic periodontitis: a systematic review. J Clin Periodontol. 2008;35(7):591–604.

Eickholz P, Kaltschmitt J, Berbig J, Reitmeir P, Pretzl B. Tooth loss after active periodontal therapy. 1: patient-related factors for risk, prognosis, and quality of outcome. J Clin Periodontol. 2008;35(2):165–74.

European Federation of Periodontology 2019. New classification of periodontal and peri-implant diseases. https://www.efp.org/fileadmin/uploads/efp/Documents/Campaigns/New_Classification/Guidance_Notes/report-02.pdf. Last accessed 22 July 2023].

Fardal Ø, Johannessen AC, Linden GJ. Tooth loss during maintenance following periodontal treatment in a periodontal practice in Norway. J Clin Periodontol. 2004;31(7):550–5.

Ferreira MC, Dias-Pereira AC, Branco-de-Almeida LS, Martins CC, Paiva SM. Impact of periodontal disease on quality of life: a systematic review. J Periodontal Res. 2017;52(4):651–65.

Foulds G, Luke DR, Teng R, Willavize SA, Friedman H, Curatolo WJ. The absence of an effect of food on the bioavailability of azithromycin administered as tablets, sachet or suspension. J Antimicrob Chemother. 1996;37(suppl C):37–44.

Genco RJ. Host responses in periodontal disease: current concepts. J Periodontol. 1992;63:338–5.

Goldman M, Ross I, Goteiner D. Effect of periodontal therapy on patients maintained for 15 years or longer. J Periodontol. 1986;57:347–53.

Griffiths GS, Ayob R, Guerrero A, Nibali L, Suvan J, Moles DR, Tonetti MS. Amoxicillin and metronidazole as an adjunctive treatment in generalized aggressive periodontitis at initial therapy or re-treatment: a randomized controlled clinical trial. J Clin Periodontol. 2011;38(1):43–9.

Guerrero A, Griffiths GS, Nibali L, Suvan J, Moles DR, Laurell L, Tonetti MS. Adjunctive benefits of systemic amoxicillin and metronidazole in non-surgical treatment of generalized aggressive periodontitis: a randomized placebo-controlled clinical trial. J Clin Periodontol. 2005;32(10):1096–107.

Gupta N, Rath SK, Lohra P. Comparative evaluation of accuracy of periodontal probing depth and attachment levels using a Florida probe versus traditional probes. Med J Armed Forces India. 2015;71(4):352–8.

Haas AN, de Castro GD, Moreno T, Susin C, Albandar JM, Oppermann RV, Rösing CK. Azithromycin as an adjunctive treatment of aggressive periodontitis: 12-months randomized clinical trial. J Clin Periodontol. 2008;35:696–704.

Haffajee AD, Socransky SS, Gunsolley JC. Systemic anti-infective periodontal therapy. A systematic review. Ann Periodontol. 2003;8(1):115–81.

Haffajee AD, Torresyap G, Socransky SS. Clinical changes following four different periodontal therapies for the treatment of chronic periodontitis: 1-year results. J Clin Periodontol. 2007;34(3):243–53.

Heasman PA, McCracken GI, Steen N. Supportive periodontal care: the effect of periodic subgingival debridement compared with supragingival prophylaxis with respect to clinical outcomes. J Clin Periodontol. 2002;29(Suppl 3):163–72; discussion 195–6

Heasman PA, Vernazza CR, Gaunt FL, Pennington MW. Cost-effectiveness of adjunctive antimicrobials in the treatment of periodontitis. Periodontol. 2011;55(1):217–30.

Hefti AF. Periodontal probing. Crit Rev Oral Biol Med. 1997;8(3):336–56.

Heitz-Mayfield LJ, Trombelli L, Heitz F, Needleman I, Moles D. A systematic review of the effect of surgical debridement vs. non-surgical debridement for the treatment of chronic periodontitis. J Clin Periodontol. 2002;29(Suppl 3):92–102; discussion 160–2

Herrera D, Sanz M, Jepsen S, Needleman I, Roldán S. A systematic review on the effect of systemic antimicrobials as an adjunct to scaling and root planing in periodontitis patients. J Clin Periodontol. 2002;29(Suppl 3):136–59; discussion 160-2

Herrera D, Alonso B, León R, Roldán S, Sanz M. Antimicrobial therapy in periodontitis: the use of systemic antimicrobials against the subgingival biofilm. J Clin Periodontol. 2008;35(8 Suppl):45–66.

Hirschfeld L, Wasserman B. A long-term survey of tooth loss in 600 treated periodontal patients. J Periodontol. 1978;49:225–37.

Hujoel PP, DeRouen TA. A survey of end point characteristics in periodontal clinical trials published 1988-92, and implications for future studies. J Clin Periodontol. 1995;22:397–407.

Hujoel PP, Loe H, Anerud A, Boysen H, Leroux BG. The informativeness of attachment loss on tooth mortality. J Periodontol. 1999;70:44–8.

Huynh-Ba G, Kuonen P, Hofer D, Schmid J, Lang NP, Salvi GE. The effect of periodontal therapy on the survival rate and incidence of complications of multirooted teeth with furcation involvement after an observation period of at least 5 years: a systematic review. J Clin Periodontol. 2009;36(2):164–76.

Kapoor A, Malhotra R, Grover V, Grover D. Systemic antibiotic therapy in periodontics. Dent Res J. 2012;9(5):505–15.

Kocher T, König J, Dzierzon U, Sawaf H, Plagmann HC. Disease progression in periodontally treated and untreated patients--a retrospective study. J Clin Periodontol. 2000;27(11):866–72.

Konig J, Plagmann H-C, Ruhling A, Kocher T. Tooth loss and pocket probing depths in compliant periodontally treated patients: a retrospective analysis. J Clin Periodontol. 2002;29:1092–100.

Lang NP, Joss A, Orsanic T, Gusberti FA, Siegrist BE. Bleeding on probing – a predictor for the progression of periodontal disease? J Clin Periodontol. 1986;13:590–6.

Lang NP, Adler R, Joss A, Nyman S. Absence of bleeding on probing – an indicator of periodontal stability. J Clin Periodontol. 1990;17:714–21.

Leininger M, Tenenbaum H, Davideau JL. Modified periodontal risk assessment score: long-term predictive value of treatment outcomes. A retrospective study. J Clin Periodontol. 2010;37(5):427–35.

Lin S, Moreinos D, Kaufman AY, Abbott PV. Tooth resorption – part 1: the evolvement, rationales and controversies of tooth resorption. Dent Traumatol. 2022;38(4):253–66.

Lindhe J, Nyman S. Long term maintenance of patients treated for advanced periodontology. J Clin Periodontol. 1984;11:504–14.

Listgarten MA. Periodontal probing: what does it mean? J Clin Periodontol. 1980;7:165–76.

Loe H, Silness J. Periodontal disease in pregnancy. (I). Prevalence and severity. Acta Odontol Scand. 1963;21:533–51.

Loe H, Anerud A, Boysen H, Morrison E. Natural history of periodontal. J Clin Periodontol. 1986;13:431–40.

Machtei EE, Hirsch I. Retention of hopeless teeth: the effect on the adjacent proximal bone following periodontal surgery. J Periodontol. 2007;78(12):2246–52.

Machtei EE, Christersson LA, Grossi SG, Dunford R, Zambon JJ, Genco RJ. Clinical criteria for the definition of "established periodontitis". J Periodontol. 1992;63(3):206–14.

Matuliene G, Pjetursson BE, Salvi GE, Schmidlin K, Bragger U, Zwahlen M, Lang NP. Influence of residual pockets on progression of periodontitis and tooth loss: results after 11 years of maintenance. J Clin Periodontol. 2008;35:685–95.

McFall WTJ. Tooth loss in 100 treated patients with periodontal disease. A long-term study. J Periodontol. 1982;53:539–49.

McGuire MK. Prognosis versus actual outcome: a long-term survey of 100 treated periodontal patients under maintenance care. J Periodontol. 1991;62:51–8.

McGuire MK, Nunn M. Prognosis vs. actual outcome. IV. The effectiveness of clinical parameters and IL-1 genotype in accurately predicting prognoses and tooth survival. J Periodontol. 1999;70:49–56.

McLeod DE, Lainson PA, Spivey JD. Tooth loss due to periodontal abscess: a retrospective study. J Periodontol. 1997;68(10):963–6.

McLeod DE, Lainson PA, Spivey JD. The predictability of periodontal treatment as measured by tooth loss: a retrospective study. Quintessence Int. 1998;29:631–5.

Miller SC. Textbook of periodontia. Philadelphia: Blakiston Co; 1950. p. 91.

Miller PD Jr. A classification of marginal tissue recession. Int J Periodontics Restorative Dent. 1985;5(2):8–13.

Nanci AT. Cate's oral histology development, structure and function. 7th ed. St. Louis: Mosby; 2008. p. 210–1.

Needleman I, McGrath C, Floyd P, Biddle A. Impact of oral health on the life quality of periodontal patients. J Clin Periodontol. 2004;31(6):454–7.

Needleman IG, Worthington HV, Giedrys-Leeper E, Tucker RJ. Guided tissue regeneration for periodontal infra-bony defects. Cochrane Database Syst Rev. 2006;19(2):CD001724.

Ng MC, Ong MM, Lim LP, Koh CG, Chan YH. Tooth loss in compliant and non-compliant periodontally treated patients: 7 years after active periodontal therapy. J Clin Periodontol. 2011;38:499–508.

Nibali L, Zavattini A, Nagata K, Di Iorio A, Lin GH, Needleman I, Donos N. Tooth loss in molars with and without furcation involvement – a systematic review and meta-analysis. J Clin Periodontol. 2016;43(2):156–66.

Nygaard-Østby P, Bakke V, Nesdal O, Susin C, Wikesjö UM. Periodontal healing following reconstructive surgery: effect of guided tissue regeneration using a bioresorbable barrier device when combined with autogenous bone grafting. A randomized-controlled trial 10-year follow-up. J Clin Periodontol. 2010;37(4):366–73.

Oteo A, Herrera D, Figuero E, O'Connor A, González I, Sanz M. Azithromycin as an adjunct to scaling and root planing in the treatment of Porphyromonas gingivalis-associated periodontitis: a pilot study. J Clin Periodontol. 2010;37(11):1005–15.

Pihlstrom BL, McHugh RB, Oliphant TH, Ortiz-Campos C. Comparison of surgical and nonsurgical treatment of periodontal disease. A review of current studies and additional results after 61/2 years. J Clin Periodontol. 1983;10(5):524–41.

Pilloni A, Rojas MA. Furcation involvement classification: a comprehensive review and a new system proposal. Dent J. 2018;6(3):34.

Polson AM. Interrelationship of inflammation and tooth mobility (trauma) in pathogenesis of periodontal disease. J Clin Periodontol. 1980;7(5):351–60.

Pretzl B, Kaltschmitt J, Kim TS, Reitmeir P, Eickholz P. Tooth loss after active periodontal therapy. 2: tooth-related factors. J Clin Periodontol. 2008;35(2):175–82.

Quirynen M, Teughels W, van Steenberghe D. Impact of antiseptics on one stage, full mouth disinfection. J Clin Periodontol. 2006;33:49–52.

Rabbani GM, Ash MM Jr, Caffesse RG. The effectiveness of subgingival scaling and root planing in calculus removal. J Periodontol. 1981;52(3):119–23.

Ramfjord SP, Caffesse RG, Morrison EC, Hill RW, Kerry GJ, Appleberry EA, Nissle RR, Stults DL. Four modalities of periodontal treatment compared over five years. J Periodontal Res. 1987a;22(3):222–3.

Ramfjord SP, Caffesse RG, Morrison EC, Hill RW, Kerry GJ, Appleberry EA, Nissle RR, Stults DL. 4 modalities of periodontal treatment compared over 5 years. J Clin Periodontol. 1987b;14(8):445–52.

Ritz L, Hefti AF, Rateitschak KH. An in vitro investigation on the loss of root substance in scaling with various instruments. J Clin Periodontol. 1991;18(9):643–7.

Sanz M, Marco Del Castillo A, Jepsen S, Gonzalez-Juanatey JR, D'Aiuto F, Bouchard P, Chapple I, Dietrich T, Gotsman I, Graziani F, Herrera D, Loos B, Madianos P, Michel JB, Perel P, Pieske B, Shapira L, Shechter M, Tonetti M, Vlachopoulos C, Wimmer G. Periodontitis and cardiovascular diseases: consensus report. J Clin Periodontol. 2020;47(3):268–88.

Silness J, Loe H. Periodontal disease in pregnancy. ii. correlation between oral hygiene and periodontal condition. Acta Odontol Scand. 1964;22:121–35.

Soares GM, Teles F, Starr JR, Feres M, Patel M, Martin L, Teles R. Effects of azithromycin, metronidazole, amoxicillin, and metronidazole plus amoxicillin on an in vitro polymicrobial subgingival biofilm model. Antimicrob Agents Chemother. 2015;59(5):2791–8.

Tonetti MS, Steffen P, Muller-Campanile V, Suvan J, Lang NP. Initial extraction and tooth loss during supportive care in a periodontal population seeking comprehensive care. J Clin Periodontol. 2000;27:824–31.

Turgut EH, Özyazici M. Bioavailability file: metronidazole. FABAD J Pharm Sci. 2004;29(1):39–49.

Walter C, Sculean A. Cone beam computed tomography (CBCT) for diagnosis and treatment planning in periodontology: a systematic review. Quintessence Int. 2016;47:25–37.

Wennström JL, Tomasi C, Bertelle A, Dellasega E. Full-mouth ultrasonic debridement versus quadrant scaling and root planing as an initial approach in the treatment of chronic periodontitis. J Clin Periodontol. 2005;32(8):851–9.

West N, Chapple I, Claydon N, D'Aiuto F, Donos N, Ide M, Needleman I, Kebschull M, British Society of Periodontology and Implant Dentistry Guideline Group Participants. BSP implementation of European S3 – level evidence-based treatment guidelines for stage I–III periodontitis in UK clinical practice. J Dent. 2021;106:103562.

Wojcik MS, DeVore CH, Beck FM, Horton JE. Retained "hopeless" teeth: lack of effect periodontally treated teeth have on the proximal periodontium of adjacent teeth 8-years later. J Periodontol. 1992;63(8):663–6.

Wood WR, Greco GW, McFall WT Jr. Tooth loss in patients with moderate periodontitis after treatment and long-term maintenance care. J Periodontol. 1989;60(9):516–20.

Abstract

This chapter discusses endodontic disease, its management and the expected outcomes of treatment. This understanding is important for the diagnosis and management of perio-endo lesions.

Endodontic Disease

Endodontic lesions occur after pulpal necrosis as a result of pulpal exposure to microbes. In the absence of treatment, this could progress to pain, infection, occasional systemic/spreading infection and eventual tooth loss. The general consensus is that tooth loss has a negative impact on quality of life, due to reduction in chewing ability following the loss of teeth (Gilbert et al. 2004; Akifusa et al. 2005; Mack et al. 2005; Baba et al. 2008; Brennan et al. 2008; Niesten et al. 2012; Wolfart et al. 2005). Reported quality of life and satisfaction outcomes of root canal treatment suggest that those with an anterior tooth that was root canal treated rather than extracted reported high satisfaction, and patients recommended preserving the natural dentition whenever possible (Dugas et al. 2002; Gatten et al. 2011).

The Diagnosis of Endodontic Disease

Most periodontal patients usually present without symptoms, and the diagnosis is based on clinical and radiographic findings, however, in endodontics, symptoms are common, and a thorough history and examination are essential for diagnosis. Accurate diagnosis and time taken to make an accurate diagnosis will be worthwhile for the patient and clinician, and may make treatment more efficient and effective. Do not underestimate the value of the patients' input into the diagnosis. Pain may only occur during the acute phases. Patients' descriptions of the symptoms, flare ups and their impression of the cause may shed light to something that is not clinically visible at the consultation visit. For example, patients may state that a certain tooth (that they can point to) was mobile when there was flare up, they may report the presence of a bad taste, which would indicate suppuration at some point, they may describe the presence of 'gum boils' and may now even have photographs on their smart phones. If a lesion recently drained or the patient has taken recent systemic antimicrobials, clinical signs may be less obvious, making diagnosis difficult.

Pain Diagnosis

A pain history should include type, intensity and frequency of the pain, stimuli and alleviating factors to enable diagnosis (Table 5.1 and Fig. 5.1). There may be a poor correlation between symptoms and the histopathological state of the pulp, however, may give some indication as to the direction of travel. For example, a throbbing aching pain that lingers, keeping the patient awake may be an indication of irreversible pulpitis, where as a sharp sensitivity that resolves when an insult is removed may indicate dentine hypersensitivity as a result of fluid movement within dentinal tubules or reversible pulpitis.

The three main primary afferent fibres in pulpal tissue are A-beta fibres (respond to light touch, normally interpreted as non-painful mechanical stimulation, but can respond as a result of inflammation, and may be affected by anti-inflammatory medication), A-delta fibres (respond to early noxious stimuli with a sharp short pain, they terminate in dentinal tubules, and therefore, can respond to fluid movement within the dentinal tubules for example with dentine hypersensitivity), and C-fibres (innervate central pulp and terminate in or beneath the odontoblast layer, therefore,

Table 5.1 A summary of pulpal status after insult

Reversible Pulpitis	Irreversible pulpitis	Necrotic pulp
Caused by mild trauma to the pulp Leads to subsequent pulpal inflammation and can cause neurogenic inflammation (sufficient mechanical damage can stimulate a nerve sprouting reaction, making the inflammation feel worse than it is) Often causes an exaggerated response to sensibility testing A-delta fibres fire as a part of normal functioning of the pulp C-fibres do not usually fire in health unless the stimulus is very intense	Vital pulp with irreversible inflammation, therefore unlikely to heal/recover Can be asymptomatic Can be very sensitive to change in temperature And is often a lingering pain, with first a sharp pain due to A-delta fibres and then a dull, less localised pain from firing C-fibres Severe inflammation can result in release of pain mediators leading to increased sensitivity of pulpal nociceptors Spontaneous pain is a clear indication of an irreversibly inflamed pulp	Non-vital tissue present in canal system Could be partially or fully non-vital May be completely asymptomatic Food source for microbes and the presence of microbes will eventually lead to inflammation or infection of the periodontal ligament

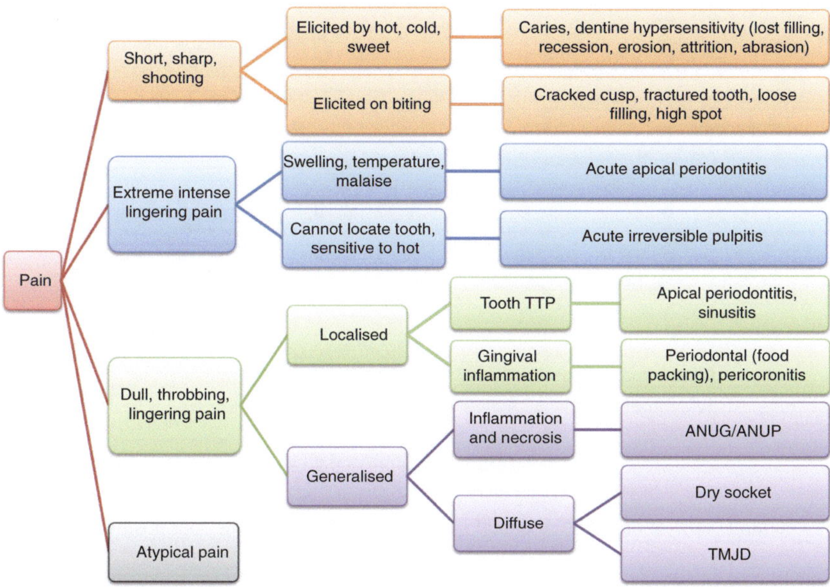

Fig. 5.1 Differential pain diagnosis

is a response to inflammation and possible tissue damage, is a late response to noxious stimuli with dull aching/burning, and pain is prolonged and intense). In the absence of tissue damage, the firing of A-delta and C-fibres is transient pain and acts as a warning. If there is tissue damage, the quality of the pain is more persistent and more intense (Hargreaves et al. 2011). With pain of periradicular origin (can be dull aching or throbbing, but should be eliminated with effective local anaesthetic), the tooth is easy to locate and the response is graded with some discomfort if percussed lightly and more discomfort if percussed heavily.

Discolouration of teeth

Grey discolouration may indicate a necrotic pulp, while a yellow discolouration may indicate tertiary dentine deposition and sclerosis. Although 4–24% of traumatised teeth develop some level of pulp canal obliteration, only 7–27% of these teeth usually develop periapical pathology, therefore, endodontic treatment is not often required pre-empting apical pathology (McCabe and Dummer 2012).

Swelling

Swelling due to periodontal disease usually occurs in the attached gingivae and rarely spreads past the mucogingival junction or leads to facial swelling. Swellings due to pulpal disease may be seen at or beyond the mucogingival junction, and may spread along the facial planes depending on the levels of muscle attachments (Fig. 5.2).

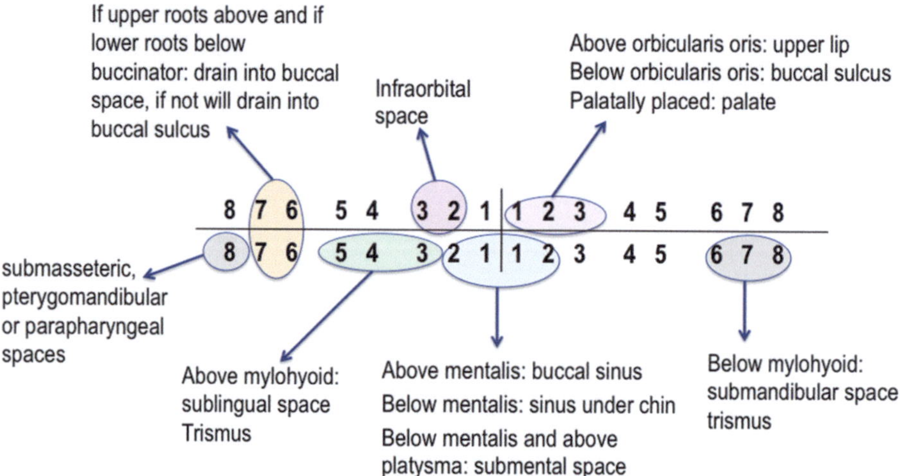

Fig. 5.2 Potential paths of drainage of dental infections depending on the root positions

Suppuration is possible with both periodontal and pulpal infection, and can be acute or chronic. Both can be draining from the gingival crevice or attached gingivae, however, in the case of infections of pulpal origin, there may be drainage from intraoral or extra oral sites. Intra oral examination may reveal swellings that are localised or diffuse, firm or fluctuant, with or without an associated sinus. Tenderness and swelling over root apices may help to identify the causative tooth when apical pathology is suspected.

Tenderness to Palpation and to Percussion (TTP)

Palpate teeth carefully with firm digital pressure over the mucosa covering the root apices. Pain on biting, palpation and tenderness on percussion indicates inflammation of the periodontal ligament (acute periradicular periodontitis) and may indicate apical pathology, however, may also indicate physical trauma/occlusal prematurities (displaying fremitus), periodontal disease or extension of pulpal disease into the periodontal ligament space. Tenderness to percussion may help to diagnose the causative tooth. Test gently with a finger, then with mirror handle. Test the contralateral tooth and adjacent teeth. Test vertically and horizontally. A negative percussion test does not however mean that the periodontal ligament space is not inflamed. Therefore, treatment should never be based on the result of one test. Numerous teeth in a quadrant that are all tender to percussion without other signs of infection may be as a result of parafunction.

Mobility

Mobility of a tooth may be as a result of parafunction, physical trauma, occlusal trauma (displaying fremitus), or as a result of periodontal disease, or due to root

Table 5.2 Reported percentage of loss of vitality under crowns and bridges

Study	Percentage of crowned teeth that lose vitality	Percentage of teeth used as bridge abutments that lose vitality
Bergenholtz and Nyman 1984: 672 initially vital teeth (255 abutments and 417 non abutments) followed up for 4-13years	3%	15%
Cheung 1991: 73 initially vital teeth observed over almost 3 years	4%	
Saunders and Saunders 1998: 458 teeth vital at the time of preparation and assessed for development of radiographic periradicular disease	19%	
Cheung et al. 2005: 122 crowns and 77 teeth as part of fixed-fixed bridges that were initially vital, followed up for 12-18 years	16%	33%

fracture, due to rapid orthodontic movement, or as a result of the extension of pulpal infection into the periodontal ligament space resulting in bone resorption and development of an apical area. Test with digital pressure on the crown in horizontal and vertical directions. Fremitus is the movement of a tooth beyond the physiological limits as a result of occlusal trauma. The tooth is usually moved out of the way before the remainder of the dentition makes contact in intercuspal position, or is the lone guiding tooth in excursions. Placing light digit pressure on the buccal aspect of the tooth in question and asking the patient to bring their teeth into occlusion and excursions can assess fremitus. If there is movement of the tooth (either seen by or felt by the examiner), the tooth can be described to be exhibiting fremitus.

Assessment of the Coronal Integrity of the Tooth

As part of the examination, the assessment of restorability is essential (Case 11), to inform treatment planning and decisions about prognosis (MtcDonad and Setchell 2005; Dawood and Patel 2017). Assessment of the coronal aspect of the tooth may also give clues as to why the tooth may have lost vitality. Between 3% and 33% of initially vital teeth develop apical pathology or lose vitality after preparation for crown and bridgework (Table 5.2).

The presence of caries, swellings, sinus, tenderness, mobility may be obvious, however assessing the presence of muscular spasm by palpating the muscles of mastication and looking for soft tissue signs of clenching and grinding, such as line alba and tongue scalloping, may give clues as to why an unrestored tooth may have lost vitality.

Periodontal Indices

As described previously, full periodontal indices (six point periodontal pocket depths, recession, bleeding, suppuration, furcation involvements and mobility) may need to follow basic periodontal examinations even in patients presenting with endodontic problems. Periodontal lesions are usually wide based and cone shaped. It is possible to track the pocket by 'stepping down' the pocket with a periodontal probe on one side of the pocket and then 'stepping up' the pocket on the other side of the pocket. Endodontic lesions draining through the periodontal pocket or near the periodontal attachment are often a narrow, deep pocket. Both lesions are usually asymptomatic, although, can develop acute exacerbations. A single deep pocket as a result of an endodontic infection tracking through or adjacent to the periodontal ligament is usually inconsistent with the level of bone loss as seen radiographically (Chapple and Lumley 1999).

Case 11 In this 68-year old female patient with less than 20% generalised horizontal bone loss, the LR6 presented with grade II mobility, a grade 1 furcation on the buccal aspect and a swelling adjacent to the furcation area in the attached gingivae (Fig. 5.3). The LR6 was minimally restored and it is not known why the LL6 was extracted (Fig. 5.4). The reason for the furcation involvement may be the presence of a furcal lateral canal or vertical fracture. The apical area indicated the need for endodontic treatment, and one should expect healing and resolution of the mobility. What would you expect the results of sensibility testing and percussion tests to be for this tooth?

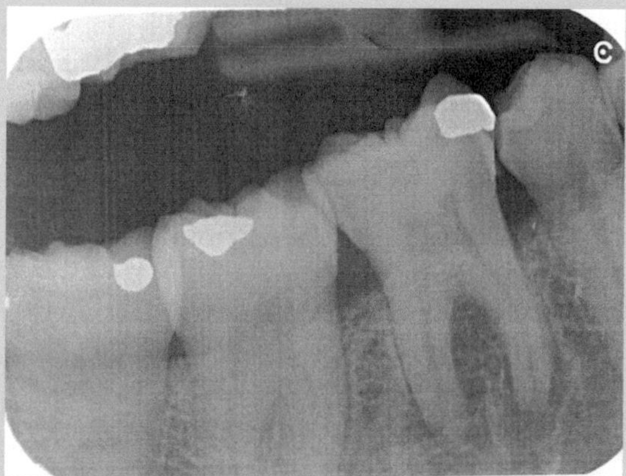

Fig. 5.3 LCPA radiograph of the LR6 showing a minimally restored LR6 with radiolucencies associated with both roots and furcation area

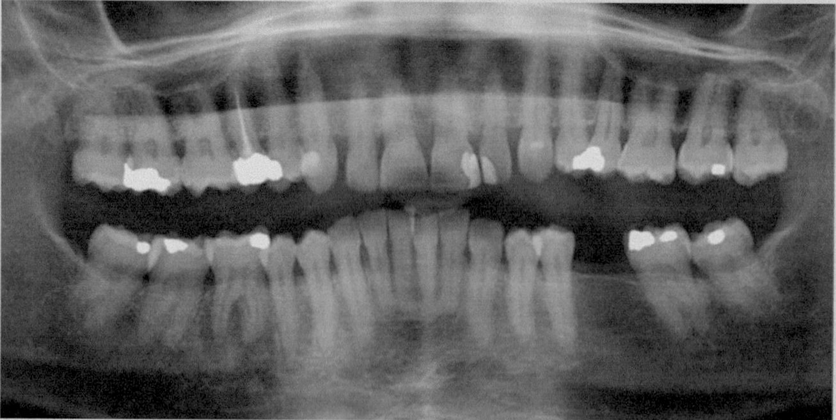

Fig. 5.4 DPT showing good general bone levels with a radiolucency associated with the minimally restored LR6 and missing LL6

Special Tests

Sensibility Testing

Sensibility testing can give an indication of the status of the pulp. All sensibility tests should have high sensitivity (ability to identify diseased teeth) and specificity (ability to identify healthy teeth). Sensibility testing can be thermal or electric (Table 5.3). Thermal testing involves the use of heat or cold to elicit a response from the pulp. A normal response is one that instantly disappears when the stimulus is removed and an abnormal response can be no response, a lingering or heightened response. Teeth that are heat sensitive may also give spontaneous pain. In some situations, patients use cold to relive pain related to irreversible pulpitis and this is an indication that pulp extirpation is necessary. In one particular case, the patient almost lost her life after months of using cold water to relieve toothache. This left the patient in neurological intensive care due to dilution hyponatraemia, followed by a seizure and encephalopathy (Porter et al. 2007).

Always test a control tooth such as the contralateral tooth first to allow the patient to understand what a normal response may feel like, and then also adjacent teeth for comparison. Isolation of the tooth being tested is important (Fig. 5.5). Repeated testing and using two different tests may give you a more accurate understanding of the status of the pulp. Although no significant differences have been shown between the use of cold testing and electric pulp testing, cold testing has been shown to be more accurate in children with less developed apices (Peters et al. 1994). A momentary or prolonged response may indicate irreversible pulpitis and no response may indicate loss of vitality. False positives may be due to partial necrosis of the pulp, or in multi-rooted teeth, when one of the canals suffering from irreversible pulpitis while another canal is infected, termed pulp necrobiosis (Grossman and Oliet 1981; Abbott and Yu 2007). Patient anxiety, ineffective isolation of the tooth (where the gingivae or saliva may conduct) and contact on metal restorations can give false negatives. False negative results may also be due to immature apices, recently traumatised teeth, contact on restorations that do not conduct, medication and high pain thresholds, as well as sclerosed canals.

Seltzer (1963) stated electric pulp testers are most accurate when there is no pulpal response to any level of electric current, meaning that 97.7% of the time a negative response to EPT indicates the need for root canal treatment (Seltzer et al. 1963a; Lin and Chandler 2008). True vitality testing requires Laser Doppler (measures velocity of blood flow) or pulse oxymetry (oxygen concentration of the blood and pulse rate) or dual wavelength spectrophotometry. Laser Doppler flowmetry is considered the most accurate of method for diagnosing the state of the pulp (Alghaithy and Qualtrough 2017). Other suggestions have been ultrasound pulse echo (uses sound) and measuring the crown surface temperature using thermographic cameras (as vital pulps are warm and re-establish their warmth quickly following cooling). A test cavity may help diagnosis; with a positive response from a pulp with vital pulp tissue, and a negative response from a pulp with pulp necrosis. It could still only show that one nerve fired and not that there there is a viable blood supply or viable pulp tissue present (Hargreaves et al. 2011). It may be difficult to

Table 5.3 Sensibility tests and their accuracy

Test	Procedure	Sensitivity (Identify diseased tooth)	Specificity (Identify healthy tooth)	Accuracy
Heat	Several possible ways: • Isolate each tooth with rubber dam, apply hot liquid from a syringe. • Use heated gutta percha (place a barrier on the tooth such as petroleum jelly to ensure the hot gutta percha does not stick to the tooth). Gutta percha warms at 65 °C, however, can warm up to 200 °C. • Dry tooth, run a dry rubber polishing wheel at high speed. A normal response is pain, increasing in intensity but decreases immediately once heat source is removed. Inflamed teeth with irreversible pulpitis will give intense immediate pain that lingers. Necrotic pulps may respond to prolonged heat as a result of remnants of the pulp fluid/gases expanding leading to pressure within the periapical region.	86%[1,2] 84–87%[3]	41%[1,2] 84–86%[3]	71%[1,2]
Cold	Use rubber dam to isolate the tooth and place • Sticks of ice. • Frozen CO_2 (dry ice/carbon dioxide snow), the temperature may be as low as −78 °C to −98 °C, therefore, protect the soft tissues. Good for teeth with crowns. • Refrigerant spray such as Endo Frost or Endo Ice (temperature of about −50 °C). The offending tooth will give no response or acute (heightened and prolonged) pain, even after the stimulus is removed. A positive response does not indicate that the pulp is not irreversibly damaged. Ethyl Chloride is not cold enough for this test.	83%[1,2] 89–94%[3]	93%[1,2] 91–93%[3]	86%[1,2]
EPT	Electric pulp testing (EPT) shows that some of the viable A-delta fibres have fired, however no information about the blood supply can be extrapolated. Some unmyelinated C-fibres may or may not respond. A false positive is possible if localised breakdown products of a necrotic pulp conduct to a viable nerve. Can be inconsistent as affected by thickness of enamel/dentine, dryness of tooth, electrical resistance of enamel presence of infractions/restorations as well as pits/fissures and caries. Ensure that teeth are separated from each other and dry (Fig 5.5). Can also be used indirectly by placing the EPT tip with a conducting medium on a probe that is placed with a conducting medium on to the tooth (useful for crowned teeth with some dentine visible). The conducting medium used is often toothpaste and some EPT machines no longer require a conducting medium. A normal pulp should respond to EPT with mild transient symptoms reversing within seconds of removing the stimulus. A positive response indicates vital pulp tissue in the coronal portion of the pulp with no information about the inflammatory status of the pulp tissue. A negative response will indicate a necrotic pulp.	72%[1,2] 75%[3]	93%[1,2] 90%[3]	81%[1,2]

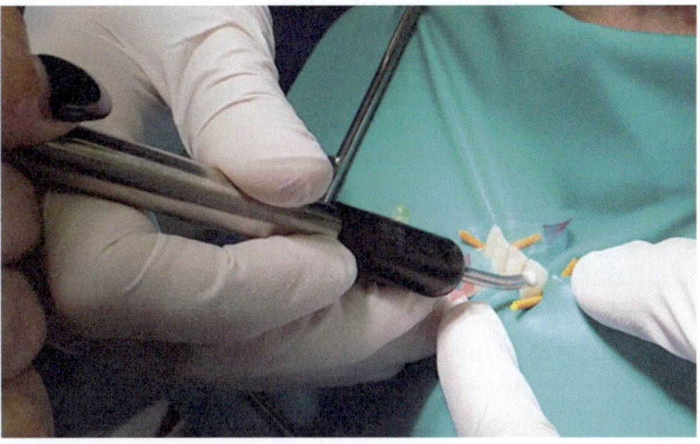

Fig. 5.5 Intra-oral photograph showing that ideally teeth should be isolated with rubber dam and separated with cellulose strips before sensibility testing to ensure each tooth responds individually

perform a test cavity in heavily restored/crowned teeth and test cavities can also give false negatives. Selective anaesthesia may have a limited use in localised diagnosis of pulpal and periodontal pathology.

> **Heat is good at telling you when a tooth is diseased**
> **Cold and EPT are good at telling you when a tooth is healthy**

Identifying Fractures

Cracked cusp syndrome was first described in 1964 (Cameron 1964). Cracked teeth have been associated with the presence of intra-coronal restorations, with mandibular second molars having the highest occurrence (Kahler 2008; Lubisich et al. 2010; Banerji et al. 2008a, b). Cracks may be identified using staining (methylene blue, and remove excess using cotton wool soaked in 70% isopropyl alcohol), transillumination, or using FractFinders/Tooth Slooth (Denbur, Oak Brook, IL, USA/ Professional Results Inc., Laguna Niguel, CA, USA). Identifying cracks within teeth may give clues to the possibility of pulpal necrosis (Fox and Youngson 1997).

When transillumination is being used, craze lines will appear as fine lines as the light is still able to pass through them, however, fractures within the tooth will prevent the light from being transmitted past the fracture line, hence the part of the tooth beyond the fracture will appear dull and grey. When FractFinders/Tooth Slooths are being used, pain on release may indicate the presence of a crack within the tooth. It must be noted that teeth that are tender to percussion due to periapical disease, can also give positive responses to FractFinders/Tooth Slooth. Orthodontic bands may be needed to identify the presence of a crack and understand the ability of the pulp to recover from the insult before cuspal coverage is provided (Eliyas et al. 2015). Vertical fractures may sometimes only be detected during surgical treatment, if not seen within the canal during root canal treatment.

Radiographic Examination

Good quality radiographs require the tooth and the roots of the tooth to be on the film, with at least 3 mm seen beyond the apex. Although it is ideal to be able to visualise the entire lesion on the radiograph, this may not be possible with long cone periapical radiographs alone. Long cone periapical radiographs are likely to give ideal images when x-ray holders are used, with the correct exposure (and for conventional radiography, when they are correctly developed). A systematic review of the literature revealed conventional plain film and digital radiographs reached the same diagnostic accuracy despite the digital technique used, with CBCT being more specific and sensitive as well as having less observer variability (Petersson et al. 2012). Radiographic appearance does not correspond to histological pathology, although, taking radiographs at different angles increases the likelihood of a correct diagnosis (Petersson et al. 2012).

Radiographic examination may not always reveal an acute infection, even with two radiographs at different angles. A periapical area may be a good indicator of periapical pathosis, however, the lack of a periapical area is not a good indicator of health. Radiographic changes may not be seen if the infection is limited to the cancellous bone or the cortical bone is of significant thickness (Rotstein and Simon 2004). In cadavers, lesions were only seen radiographically when they invaded the junction between the cancellous and cortical bone (Bender et al. 1961). Where there is thin cortical bone and the roots are closer to the junction between the cortical plate and the cancellous bone (such as anterior teeth), lesions may be seen earlier than where the roots are further away from the junction (such as palatal roots of maxillary molars or roots of mandibular molars). A lesion needs to break the cortex or significantly erode the inside of the cortex to be visible on radiographs. If there is a draining sinus present, the placement of a gutta percha (GP) point into the draining sinus prior to taking a radiograph will allow better understanding of the origin of the infection (Fig. 5.6a–c). Extra orally, draining sinuses may also lend themselves to placement of GP points (Fig. 5.7a–d). In maxillary teeth swellings/sinuses may present buccally or palatally, and although lingual swellings are possible with

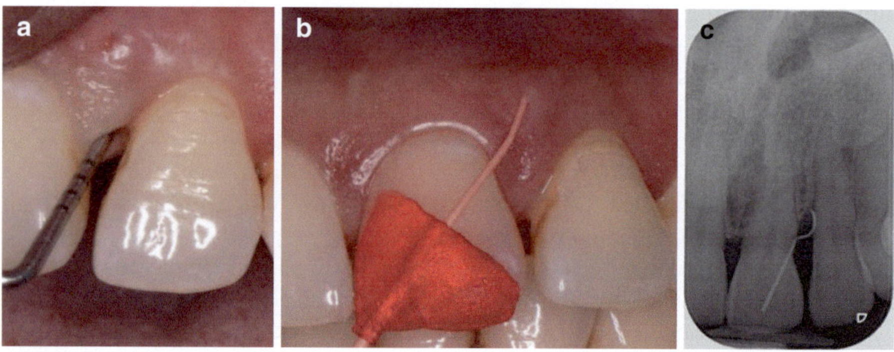

Fig. 5.6 Intra-oral photographs and LCPA radiographs of the UL2: The use of a GP point in any draining sinus present can help to identify the source of the infection (**a**). A gutta percha point (#25) secured in situ with ribbon wax on a dry tooth (**b**), and the excess gutta percha beyond the occlusal surface of the tooth is cut to avoid the patient biting on it and moving the gutta percha point before taking a LCPA radiograph (**c**). (Picture courtesy of Mr. Vithurran Vijayenthiran)

mandibular teeth, sinuses do not often drain lingually. Sometimes, sinus tracts are lined with epithelium, although frequently they are lined with granulation tissue, and most heal when the cause is treated.

The utilisation of small volume CBCTs have been recommended in endodontics. The use of which should follow thorough clinical and plain film radiographic examination. CBCT should only be used when additional information is likely to aid diagnosis or clinical management, such as assessment of the extent of resorption defects, complex anatomy like dens invaginatus, the presence of fractures or perforations, the search for missed or sclerosed canals and extent of large apical lesions when surgery is being considered (Patel et al. 2019; European Society of

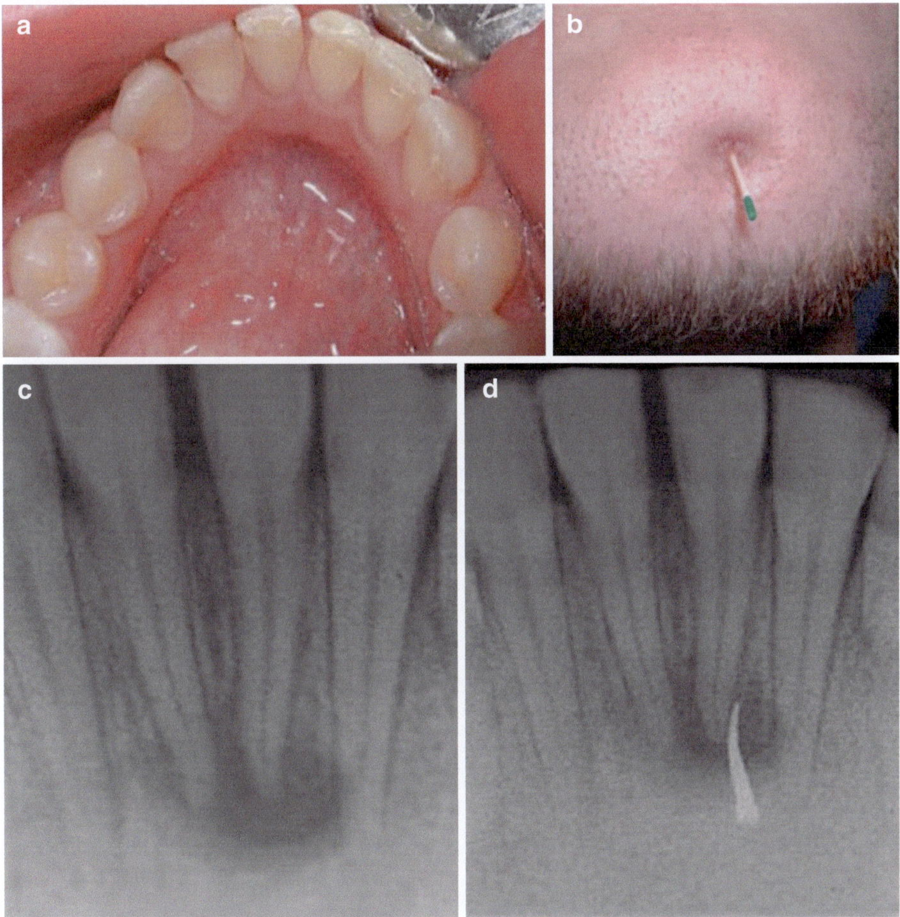

Fig. 5.7 Intra-oral and extra-oral photographs and LCPA radiographs of the lower anterior mandible: An extra orally draining sinus as a result of non-vital lower central incisor teeth (**a** and **b**), which clinically look sound. LCPA radiographs of the lower central incisors show the presence of apical periodontitis (**c**) and the GP point tracked to the LL1 (**d**). (Pictures courtesy of Mr. Peter Briggs)

Endodontology 2019). The presence of an apical area on the CBCT, post endodontic treatment, does not mean that the area is not healing. As technology improves, the dose of CBCTs may reduce significantly, and the benefit of three-dimensional viewing may outweigh the dose.

Extensive fractures may be visible on radiographs (Fig. 5.8), and smaller fractures may occasionally be seen on plain film radiographs depending on whether x-ray beam is within 4 degrees of the fracture plane (i.e. root fractures can only be seen on a radiograph if the x-ray beam almost passes through the fracture line). Fractures could be visible on CBCT (Rotstein and Simon 2004). In periodontally sound dentitions, single vertical defects may be indicative of a fracture. 'Halo' like, 'J' shaped or isolated vertical bone loss around a tooth may indicate the presence of a fracture. A fracture from the mesial to the distal of a tooth may appear as an abnormal widening of the periodontal ligament. Endodontic issues related to fractures within teeth may be difficult to differentiate from periodontal disease and true perio-endo lesions. In the absence of 'halo' like or 'J' shaped lesions, vertical root fractures can also appear as a widened periodontal ligament, as also seen with occlusal trauma. Clinically, localised bone loss and a deep periodontal pocket is seen when the fracture is long standing.

Table 5.4 summarises the clinical and radiographic signs to consider when suspecting pathology of endodontic origin. As can be seen, some of these endodontic signs are those that would also be seen in periodontal pathology.

Fig. 5.8 LCPA radiograph of the UR4. A fracture in the UR4 appears as a mesial vertical bone defect. Due to the angulation of the radiation beam in relation to the fracture, the fracture is visible

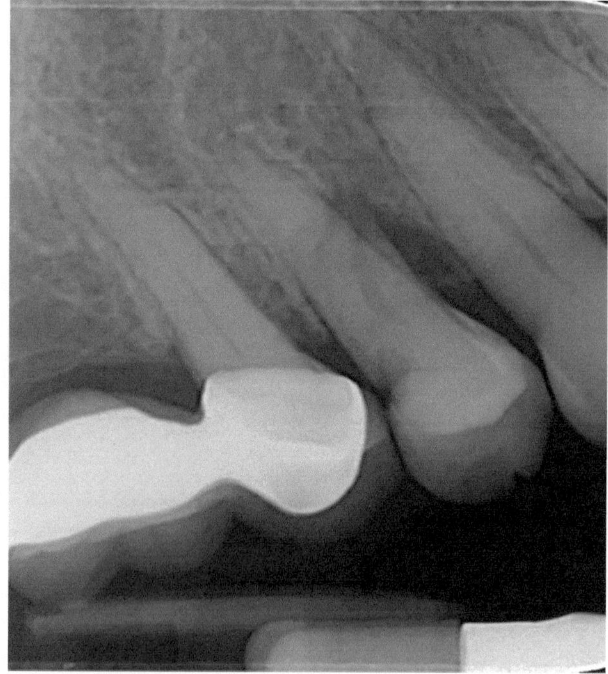

Table 5.4 A summary of clinical and radiographic signs to be aware of during examination

Pain History	Visual examination	Radiographic examination
Type: Sharp or dull/throbbing or steady **Intensity:** mild/moderate/severe **Frequency:** intermittent/constant **Stimuli:** heat/cold or pressure **Relieving factors:** cold or pressure **Location:** can patient identify causative tooth	Presence and location of swelling: attached gingivae/ mucogingival junction/ spreading along facial planes Presence of suppuration Presence and shape of periodontal pockets Mobility: test vertically and horizontally Percussion test Palpation over the root apices for swelling and tenderness Sensibility testing	Place GP point in any sinus tracts present: –If tracking to apex of tooth, likely to be due to pulpal pathology –If tracking to mid-root, furcation or any other part of the root, suspect lateral canal or periodontal involvement (Sistla *et al.* 2018)

The Treatment of Endodontic Disease

The wider management of endodontic disease would involve the prevention of dental disease and trauma that may lead to necrosis of the pulp tissue. However, once pulp vitality has been lost, ideally before infection, the objective of endodontic treatment is to clean and seal the root canal system, both apically and coronally such that there is no entry of microbes into the root canal system, and there is no space left within the root canal system for the cultivation of bacteria. The goals of chemo-mechanical root canal preparation have been described as removal of vital/necrotic tissue from the main canal system, creation of sufficient space for irrigation and medication, preservation of the integrity and location of the apical anatomy, avoiding iatrogenic damage to the canal system/root structure, facilitation of canal filling, avoiding further contamination of the periradicular tissues with irrigants/infection whilst reserving sound tooth structure (Hülsmann et al. 2005; Schilder 1974). In the infected tooth, this also involves the removal of as much of the microbes as possible from the root canal system, along with the previous root canal filling, if previously root filled. It is not recommended that potentially infected debris be forced beyond the apical foramen (Schilder 1974; Ricucci and Langeland 1998).

Over 30 years ago, it was shown that when strict protocols for removing bacteria were used by undergraduates, and strict criteria of success were being used to assess the outcome of root filled teeth, the presence and absence of apical pathology influences the outcome (Sjogren 1990). The findings are summarised in Table 5.5.

Sjogren (1990) showed that instrumenting to the apical constriction influences periapical healing for necrotic teeth that were not previously root canal treated, with only 69% healing if not instrumented to the apical constriction compared to 90% healing if instrumented to the apical constriction. This difference was less significant with previously root filled teeth with apical areas present (Sjogren 1990). In vital cases, excess root filling had no impact on outcome, possibly as a result of the inert root filling being uninfected, although present in the apical tissues (Sjogren 1990). The measurement of the apical constriction at that time was carried out using radiographs, however, more recent studies have shown achievement of patency (now using apex locators) to be important (Ng et al. 2011a).

Table 5.5 The success of root canal treatment has been long associated with the status of the pulp and the presence or absence of peri-apical pathology (Sjogren et al. 1990)

Pulp status	Vital pulp	Necrotic pulp		Previously failed root canal treatment	
Periapical status	No periapical area	No periapical area	Periapical area present	No periapical area	Periapical area present
Success	96%	98%	86%	Not reported	62%

Table 5.6 The factors that determine the success of root canal treatment (Ng et al. 2011a; Sjogren 1990)

Pre-operative factors	Peri-operative factors	Post-operative factors
• The presence of periapical lesion reduces the odds of success by 49% • The presence of periapical lesion with success being reduced by 4% for every 1mm of increase in size of the lesion • The presence of a pre-operative sinus tract reduces the odds of success by 48% • The presence of a root perforation reduces the odds of success by 56%	• Achievement of patency at the canal terminus increases the likelihood of success by two fold • Extension of canal cleaning as close as possible to its apical terminus. Short root fillings reduce the odds of success by 12% for every 1mm short of the apex and extrusion of the root filling material reduces the odds of success by 62% • The use of EDTA solution as a penultimate wash followed by a final rinse of NaOCl in root canal re-treatment cases increases the odds of success by two-fold • The use of 0.2% CHX as an adjunctive irrigant to NaOCl solution reduces the odds of success by 53% • Inter-appointment flare-ups reduce the odds of success by 47%	• The presence of satisfactory coronal restoration increases the odds of success by 11 fold.

Vital cases should be treated via a biological approach. The pulp may be inflamed, causing pain, and therefore, removal of the inflamed portion of the pulp (pulpotomy) or removal of the whole pulp (pulpectomy) may be required. It is possible not to instrument to the apical constriction and still avoid developing apical periodontitis, however, the most important aspect is not to introduce bacteria into the canal system. In vital cases partial instrumentation may lead to increased pain, and patients should be warned of this.

Non-vital cases without infection can be treated somewhat like vital cases; however, all of the non-vital tissue must be removed. Non-vital cases with infection should be treated via a microbiologically based approach. Pain in these non-vital cases may be related to an imbalanced host-parasite relationship, and communication of the pulp chamber with the oral environment. The aim of the first stage of endodontic should be the complete removal of the necrotic tissue, preparation to the working length and copious irrigation to reduce the bacterial load. In re-treatment (or secondary root canal treatment) cases, one should aim to understand the reasons for failure, in order to correct them as part of the re-treatment. Often the cause of failure is the presence or ingress of microbes, therefore, all of the previous root canal filling must be removed and chemo-mechanical cleaning performed. Careful examination under an operating microscope may reveal other reasons for failure such as fractures within the root. The outcome of endodontics has been correlated with a number of pre-operative, peri-operative and post-operative factors and can be seen in Table 5.6 (Ng et al. 2011a).

Recommended protocols for endodontic treatment include the following (European Society of Endodontology 2006):

1. **Pre-operative radiographic assessment**: The use of diagnostic quality radiographs that allow visualisation of at least the full length of the root and approximately 2–3 mm the periapical region, to be able to picture the full extent of any periradicular pathology, are recommended. An estimation of the length from the cusp tip (to be used as the reference point) to the pulp chamber, using a bitewing radiograph (most parallel radiograph) is appropriate for posterior teeth. An estimation of the full length of the root and root morphology using a long cone periapical radiograph is essential.

2. **Local anaesthesia** should be considered and given as appropriate.

3. **Removal of existing restorations:** All caries and defective restorations should be removed, and if required, the occlusion adjusted as well as the tooth protected against fracture. The removal of restoration will reveal potential leakage, fractures, and caries, as well as allow determination of the prognosis and ability to provide a predictable restoration after root canal treatment. When 254 teeth were assessed for the presence of marginal leakage using clinical and radiographic parameters and then compared to the findings after dismantling the restorations, it was found that there was only a 56% chance of detecting caries, cracks or marginal breakdown prior to restoration removal. When the restorations were removed, 95% of the teeth had one or more factors that could have contributed to pulpal and periapical disease (Abbott 2004).

4. **Isolation** using rubber dam is essential for patient safety (Heling and Heling 1977; Silva et al. 2011; Ahmad 2009) and better endodontic outcomes (Van Nieuwenhuysen et al. 1994; Ahmad 2009). Rubber dam can take less than 2 minutes to apply (Heise 1971; Cunningham and Ferguson 1970) and is well tolerated by patients (Reuter 1983; Stewardson and McHugh 2002). The use of an appropriate caulking agent is recommended (Fig. 5.9).

5. **Access cavity preparation** should include the remove roof of the pulp chamber, enabling root canal instruments to enter the canal without undue bending and offer sufficient retention for a temporary restoration, conserving as much

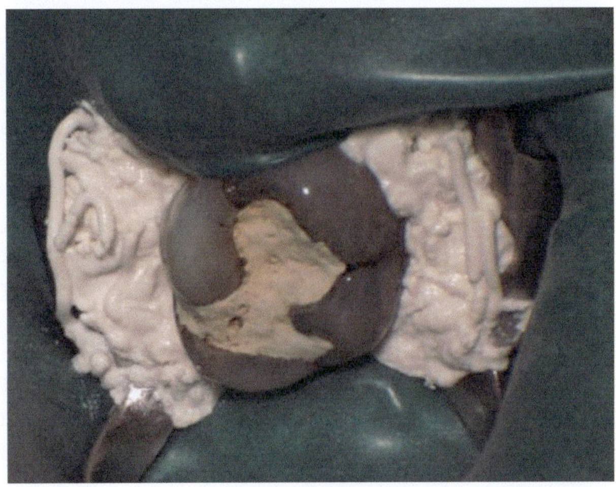

Fig. 5.9 Use of caulking agents

sound tooth structure as possible. The crown-down technique (Fairbourn et al. 1987) is recommended, where orifice opening, coronal flare and preparation to two-thirds of the estimated length of the canal is completed before accessing the apical third, because the majority of the microbes are likely to be present in the coronal and mid third of the pulp canal system. Removal of coronal bacteria avoids contamination of the more apical pulpal (potentially non-infected) tissues (Shovelton 1964; Haapasalo et al. 2005; Huang et al. 2015; Young et al. 2007). The prepared canal should include the original canal as well as maintain the original shape of the canal. The apical constriction should be kept as small as possible and maintained in its original position. The preparation should end at the apical narrowing with the canal tapering from the crown to the apex. This is in order to maintain the biological objectives of confining the instrumentation to within the root canal, removal of all of the tissue from the root canal space, creation of sufficient space for intracanal medicaments and not forcing necrotic and potentially infected debris beyond the foramen (Schilder 1974).

6. **Irrigation**: Copious irrigation is recommended, with a solution that has disinfectant and organic debris dissolving properties, extending as far apical as possible in the canal without risking extrusion beyond the foramen. Irrigation may be activated/delivered by ultrasonic or sonic systems (Cheung et al. 2021). Mechanical debridement cannot be relied upon to remove a significant portion of infected dentine due to the complexity of the root canal system. Studies have shown that between 31–57% of the main canal can be left untouched by root canal instruments (Peters et al. 2001; Silveira et al. 2010; Paqué et al. 2010, 2011). Passing instruments through a reservoir of irrigant to reduce the likelihood of microbial contamination of the more apical pulpal tissue is good practice.

   The safe use of irrigants requires small gauge (28–30), side exit needles, measured and bent to 3–4 mm short of the estimated working length (Eliyas et al. 2010). The irrigant flows only 1 mm beyond the tip of the needle (Hülsmann et al. 2007) and therefore, when the apex locator zero reading has been established, the length of the needle measurement can be revised to 1–2 mm short of the working length (bearing in mind the size of the apical third to allow reverse flow of the irrigant, and the size of the apical foramen to prevent extrusion). Smaller gauge needles (gauge 30) have been shown to cause less extrusion of irrigant beyond the canal (Uzunoglu-Özyürek et al. 2017).

   Although many different irrigants have been suggested (Zehnder 2006; Haapasalo et al. 2005; Jena et al. 2015), Sodium hypochlorite is the irrigant of choice as it is able to both dissolve organic material (at concentrations higher than 1%) and is bactericidal at concentrations over 0.5% (Estrela et al. 2002; Bystrom and Sundqvist 1983; Radcliffe et al. 2004; Sirtes et al. 2005). 1% sodium hypochlorite warmed in a baby bottle bath to 45 °C can be as effective as using 5.25% at 20 °C, as higher temperatures release more chlorine molecules, with 100% of the chlorine being available for at least 60 minutes (Sirtes et al. 2005). Higher concentration may be thicker and subsequently cause less wetting of the dentinal walls (Bonsor et al. 2006) and may cause more damage if extruded through the apex or perforations into soft tissues. All concentrations above 0.5% can degrade collagen in dentine (Driscoll et al. 2002). Some have advocated prolonged contact time in the canal (of up to 40 minutes) to be effective (Spangberg et al. 1973). For some microbes such as *Enterococcus faecalis* to be undetectable, contact periods of up to 30 minutes of soaking in sodium hypochlorite maybe required, depending on the concentration (Bonso et al. 2006).

Sodium hypochlorite does not remove inorganic material, and therefore, the use of EDTA, a chelating agent, usually in liquid form of 15–17%, is required for smear layer removal. EDTA, although not bactericidal or bacteriostatic, can chelate metallic ions, starving microbes and inhibiting their growth (Seidberg and Schilder 1974; Nygaard-Østby 1957). EDTA removes calcium leaving a softened matrix of dentine, emulsifies soft tissue without deleterious effect to pulpal or periapical tissues (Nygaard-Østby 1957). The active molecules in these irrigants are self-limiting, and therefore, frequent changing of the irrigant solution within the canal is required, however, excessive use (17% for more than 10 minutes) can erode peritubular and intertubular dentine (Calt and Serper 2002). For the desired effect, EDTA may need to be in the canal system for 1–5 minutes (Weinreb and Meier 1965; Hülsmann et al. 2003), and soaking the canal for 1, 3 and 5 minutes have been shown to be equally effective at removing the smear layer (Teixeira et al. 2005). Dynamic pulping or activation of the irrigant with ultrasonic may be beneficial (Ng et al. 2011a).

7. **Working length and first binding file**: The ideal method of finding the physiological foramen at the end of a root is histological analysis, which is not clinically possible. Other methods include patient response to pain, tactile sense of the operator, paper point technique (where a dry, well fitting paper point is placed in the canal, then removed from the canal to measure from the wet part of the paper point to a reference point to give some estimation of the length of the canal, which can be useful in open apex or canals with apical resorption), radiographs and electronic apex locators. The later two being more accurate than the former three options. The working length should be as close to the apical constriction as possible, i.e. between 0.5 and 2 mm of the radiographic apex (Sjogren et al. 1990; Ng et al. 2011a). The use of electronic and radiographic methods to determine the working length has been recommended.

The accuracy of radiographs for working length measurement has been reported to be between 64% and 76% (Real et al. 2011; Bahrololoomi et al. 2015), with it sometimes being necessary to take more than one working length radiograph. Electronic apex locators, especially third, fourth and fifth generation, are considered to be very accurate at informing when the file is just outside the canal. Numerous studies have compared electronic apex locators, radiographs to histological and micro-CT images of the major foramen. Electronic apex locators have been found to be to be more than 90% accurate at identifying the apical constriction, with some models being better than others, as well as being more accurate the closer the instrument is to the physiological constriction (Real et al. 2011; Silveira et al. 2011; Bahrololoomi et al. 2015; Gordon and Chandler 2004). The use of a smooth file such as a finger spreader (so as not to disturb the apex) and a file that is closer to the natural size of the canal will produce a more accurate result (Shacham et al. 2020). Apex locators appear to be less accurate at identifying the major foramen, leading to overestimation of the working length and instrumentation beyond the apical foramen (Connert et al. 2018). The differences between apex locator reading and the physiological apical constriction is <0.5 mm, and is of no clinical significance due to the manual ability of any operator. Over instrumentation may have an impact on histological healing.

When using an apex locator, it is advised that the apex locator zero reading (when the instrument is just outside the canal) be used to then calculate the working length, which may be 0.5 or 1 mm short of the apex locator zero reading (Ricucci 1998; Ricucci and Langeland 1998; Sjogren et al. 1990; Ng et al. 2011a). More accurate apex locator readings are possible when the coronal and mid-flare have already been completed, debris removed, and foramen not enlarged. Shaping of the more coronal aspects of the canal and removing and interferences can make estimation of the first binding file more accurate (Silveira et al. 2008). Most electronic apex locators now tend to be accurate with the use of sodium hypochlorite, and some to a lesser degree with EDTA as a medium within the canal. Electronic apex locator readings can be inaccurate with immature roots, damaged periodontal ligaments, in the presence of metal restorations, caries, saliva, bleeding and exudate at the apex, and with mediums of extreme conducting properties such as distilled water or saline. Identification of the first binding file in the apical third by tactile sense when establishing the apex locator zero reading will also allow a decision to be made as to whether the canal requires further enlarging. In true perio–endo lesions, it may be imperative that apical instrumentation of the whole canal is achieved and therefore accurate working length calculation is important (Baugh and Wallace 2005).

8. **Preparation of the apical third of the canal** should allow irrigation to reach the full working length and create a tapered preparation that is easy to fill, whilst retaining as much of the dentine as possible. This can be achieved with hand or rotary instruments, the latter of which, may be more efficient with better maintenance of the canal shape (Haapasalo et al. 2005). Initially, it was taught that canals should be prepared to three sizes above the first binding file (Weine 1989), however, now a more microbiological approach is advocated with canal preparation to allow entry of irrigant to the working length (Khademi et al. 2006) and avoid extrusion in the tissues beyond the apex of the root (Uzunoglu-Özyürek et al. 2017). It is accepted that the apical stop created is an International Organisation for Standardisation (ISO) size 25–30 to allow irrigants to reach the apical third and still preserve a maximal amount of dentine (Yared and Dagher 1994; Khademi et al. 2006; Uzunoglu-Özyürek et al. 2017). Canals are rarely circular and therefore, either the largest diameter needs to be prepared to, or accept that some areas of the apical area remains uninstrumented. The latter may be the more sensible approach as over preparation can damage the apical foramen and lead to strip perforations (Silveira et al. 2008;

Baugh and Wallace 2005). Apical gauging before obturation is recommended. It is wise to ensure the following details in are recorded in the clinical notes:

Isolation: Rubber dam and use of caulking agent
Irrigation: 17% EDTA and 1% Sodium hypochlorite warmed to 40°c
Activation of irrigant: Ultrasonic or mastercone GP point and dynamic pumping

Canal	Ref Point	Estimated working length	Apex Locator Zero	Working Length	1st binding file	Patency gained and maintained	Prepared Size	Apical Gauge

9. **Inter-appointment medication**: Inter-appointment medication should be used following proper cleaning and irrigation, and to support the tissue dissolving effects of the irrigating solutions. The medicament used should have long lasting disinfection properties, be biocompatible, removable and non-damaging to the tooth structure or restorative material. When using multiple visits to complete treatment leave at least 5–7 days between appointments to allow the periradicular tissues to recover and to maximise the antimicrobial effect of intracanal medications such as calcium hydroxide. It is not possible to completely fill and seal the apical portion of root canal systems (Oliver and Abbott 2001), however, it may be possible to alter the environment of the canal system towards that which is unfavourable for bacterial colonisation using intracanal medicaments for the duration of the periodontal treatment in perio-endo lesions (Tronstad et al. 1987, 1990; Abbott 1990a, b). This may help prevent bacterial entry from the periodontium into the canal system during healing.

Chemo-mechanical cleaning alone may not necessarily render a root canal system free of bacteria, however, inter-appointment dressing with calcium hydroxide may do so (Zehnder et al. 2002). Calcium hydroxide has initially bactericidal and then bacteriostatic properties, and has also been thought to have healing properties that encourage bony healing (Cheung 2002; Ba-Hattab et al. 2016; Kim and Kim 2014; Kim and Kim 2015). Calcium hydroxide stimulates hard tissue repair, but also causes necrosis due to high toxicity and this may aggravate inflammation. In cases where the cementum has been removed, calcium hydroxide seeping out of the dentinal tubules may lead to initiation or exacerbation of external inflammatory root resorption, therefore, long term use of calcium hydroxide may be associated with ankylosis (Pierce et al. 1988; Pierce and Lindskog 1987; Vernillo et al. 1994; Lengheden et al. 1991a, b; Blomlöf et al. 1992; Solomon et al. 1995). Ledermix paste (Lederle Laboratories, Seefeld, Germany), a corticosteroid-antibiotic combination with an anti-inflammatory effect, has been recommended to reduce periodontal and periapical inflammation. It has been suggested that a mixture of both Ledermix and Calcium hydroxide may be better for preventing resorption (Abbott and Salgado 2009). Tetracyclines have also been suggested as an inter-appointment dressing because they bind to bone and tooth, and this binding may keep the medicament in the local region for sufficient time to allow periodontal healing (Abbott and Salgado 2009).

Healing of the sinus tract is usually rapid, and may heal between appointments, however, depending on the chronicity, may require multiple appointments and may take 3–6 months to heal (Simon et al. 1972). If attempting to prevent resorption, the dressing needs to be replaced at regular intervals. This stage is not necessary in vital cases and those that can be completed in one visit. No difference in outcome has been found when comparing single-visit endodontics with multiple visits (Field et al. 2004; Figini et al. 2008; Singh and Garg 2012; Paredes-Vieyra and Enriquez 2012; Friedman 2002; Weiger et al. 2000; Peters and Wesselink 2002). Therefore, even infected teeth can heal with one visit endodontics. It is not known if this could also be extrapolated to perio–endo lesions.

10. **Inter-appointment restoration**: An effective temporary restoration is essential to prevent contamination of canals between visits. A 'double seal' with sponge over the canal orifices, Cavit or Coltasol (Coltene Whaldent, Mahwah, NJ, USA) and IRM (Dentsply Caulk, Milford, USA) have been recommended because they are easy to place and remove, cheap, and form a good seal between appointments. In the case of teeth requiring a post to retain a core, it would be better to restore the root with a double seal and then provide a denture to replace the coronal tooth structure until the root canal treatment can be completed and the definitive post and core be placed (Naoum and Chandler 2002; Eliyas et al. 2015).

11. **Obturation of the canal system** should use materials that are biocompatible, dimensionally stable, able to seal, unaffected by tissue fluids and insoluble, non-supportive of bacterial growth, radio-opaque, and removable from the canal if re-treatment is needed. The objective of obturation is to provide and coronal seal against microbes and nutrients entering the canal system, provide an apical seal against nutrients entering from the apical tissues and to entomb any remaining microbes within the canal system (Tomson et al. 2014). A sealer must be used to fill the voids between a semi-solid filling material and the walls of the canal. Sealers containing organic materials such as aldehydes are not recommended due to carcinogenicity, although the quantity released from endodontic material is small (Athanassiadis et al. 2015). Obturation should follow chemo-mechanical debridement and preparation (when the canal is thought to be free of infection and can be dried), and after a radiograph verifying the preparation has been taken (a master-cone radiograph where gutta percha is used and a mid-fill radiograph where mineral trioxide aggregate, MTA, is used). Obturating to within 2 mm of the radiographic apex, and staying within the canal have been shown to lead to better outcomes (Sjogren 1990; Ng et al. 2011a). Gutta percha in the floor of the pulp chamber must be removed, as it does not provide an adequate seal, especially in multi-rooted teeth where furcal/accessory canals may be present (Rotstein and Simon 2004).

12. **Post-operative radiographic examination**: The quality of the filling must be checked with a post-operative radiograph, which should show the root apex and preferably 2–3 mm of the periapical region. The obturated canal should be completely filled (without voids) unless a post space is required, and contain the original

canal. No space should be seen between the canal filling and the canal walls. There should be no canal space visible beyond the end point of the root canal filling.

13. **Post operative restoration of the tooth:** Coronal leakage can lead to failure of endodontic treatment (Madison and Wilcox 1988; Ray and Trope 1995; Saunders and Saunders 1994); therefore, provision of a definitive coronal seal as soon as possible after completion of endodontic treatment is recommended, with provision of a cuspal coverage restoration for posterior teeth with suspicion of cracks or breaching of the marginal ridges (Torabinerjad et al. 1990; Ng et al. 2011a; Rotstein and Simon 2004). The time of crown placement has been correlated with survival, with teeth that were crowns more than 4 months after completion of root canal treatment being three times as likely to undergo extraction when compared to teeth that were crowned within 4 months of completion of endodontic treatment (Pratt et al. 2016).

14. **Re-assessment of healing** should be assessed at least after 1 year after treatment completion, and subsequently as required for 'favourable outcome' (absence of pain, swelling and other symptoms, absence of a sinus tract, no loss of function and radiological evidence of a normal periodontal ligament around the root), 'uncertain outcome' (periapical lesion remains the same size or has only reduced in size). In this situation it is recommended that the lesion be further monitored for a minimum period of 4 years (Strindberg 1956; Del Fabbro et al. 2007). If the lesion persists, the tooth may be associated with post-treatment disease and be deemed to have an 'unfavourable outcome' (tooth is associated with signs and symptoms of infection, a radiologically visible lesion has appeared subsequent to treatment or a pre-existing lesion has increased in size, the lesion has remained the same size or only diminished slightly in size during the 4-year assessment period, or continuing root resorption is present). The exception is the presence of scar tissue (an extensive radiological lesion may heal but leave a locally visible, irregularly mineralised area) and required continued review (Nair 2006).

Surgical Endodontic Treatment

Surgical endodontic treatment should only be considered for failed cases when non-surgical endodontic treatment has been provided, and the canal system has been cleaned, obturated and sealed to the best of one's ability. Many have described the techniques for endodontic microsurgery (Von Arx et al. 2019; Eliyas et al. 2014; Kim and Kratchman 2006). In terms of the outcomes of surgical endodontics, outcomes are better if non-surgical endodontic treatment is completed before surgical treatment, and outcomes are poorer when there is poor access for surgery, persisting lesions despite an apparent good root canal filling, when the size of the lesion exceeds 5 mm, when there is coronal leakage and when surgical re-treatment is performed (Tsesis et al. 2013). Do not judge the quality of the endodontic treatment purely on the appearance of the root filling seen radiographically, as the way in which the treatment was performed is unknown. Although, there is evidence to suggest that the outcome of endodontic treatment is better if the root filling as seen radiographically, is filled to within 2 mm of the radiographic apex, has good taper and no voids present (Ng et al. 2011a; Farzaneh et al. 2004). The use of rubber dam, adequate irrigation and maintaining patency is not ascertainable from the radiograph, yet will impact outcome (Ng et al. 2011a). It is possible that a seemingly well-filled root canal filing may harbour bacteria, and therefore, if there are doubts surrounding the possibility of endodontic infection, non-surgical endodontic retreatment should be attempted, before considering surgical endodontics. Like that for periodontal treatment, the outcome of endodontic treatment is better in the first year for surgical treatment, however at 4 years the differences between surgical and non-surgical treatment become less significant. This is accounted for by late failures in the surgical group and the prolonged time required for healing of some lesions in the non-surgical group (Del Fabbro et al. 2007).

The Outcome of Endodontic Treatment

Outcomes of root canal treatment have previously been studied and assessed by clinicians and researchers using radiographs, clinical signs and symptoms (Friedman et al. 2002; Ng et al. 2007), as it is neither practical nor ethical to have histological sections, although these would allow definite outcomes of healing to be assessed. Patients will measure outcome in relation to the absence of symptoms (Bender et al. 1966a, b), function and aesthetics (Friedman and Mor 2004) and overall quality of life (Dugas et al. 2002; Gatten et al. 2011; Hamasha and Hatiwsh 2013).

As can be seen from Tables 5.7 and 5.8, root canal treatment and maintenance of the natural tooth has high success rates (Ng et al. 2011a) and high survival rates (Lazarski et al. 2001; Salehrabi and Rotstein 2004; Chen et al. 2007; Torabinejad et al. 2007; Lumley et al. 2008; Tickle et al. 2008; Ng et al. 2010, 2011b), with fewer interventions than implant-supported prostheses (Doyle et al. 2006). Studies have reported no significant difference in the survival rates of root filled teeth and of implant-supported single crowns (Torabinejad et al. 2007; Doyle et al. 2006, 2007; Iqbal and Kim 2007; Hannahan and Eleazer 2008; Morris et al. 2009). Survival rates of implants provided by inexperienced practitioners is reported as being approximately 20% lower than that provided by specialists in implant placement (Morris

Table 5.7 A systematic review comparing the various options summarised the weighted success and survival rates of implant-supported single crowns, bridgework and root filled teeth (Torabinejad et al. 2007)

	Success			Survival		
	2–4 years	4–6 years	6+ years	2–4 years	4–6 years	6+ years
Implant-supported single crown	99%	98%	95%	96%	97%	97%
Fixed-partial dentures (bridges)	78%	76%	80%	94%	93%	82%
Root filled teeth	89%	94%	84%	94%	94%	97%

Table 5.8 Survival and success rates for endodontic treatment (primary root canal treatment is when a tooth has undergone root canal treatment for the first time and secondary endodontic treatment is when revision root canal treatment or re-treatment has been provided)

Survival rates		Success rates	
Lazarski *et al.* 2001 (109,542 teeth, data collected over 5 years)	94.4% at 3.5 years	Success rate of primary root canal treatment (Ng *et al.*2007) Pooled weighted success from 63 studies assessed	74.7% using 'strict' criteria in 40 studies (95% CI: 69.8%, 79.5%) 85.2% using 'loose' criteria in 36 studies (95% CI: 82.2%, 88.3%)
Salehrabi & Rotstein 2004 (1,462,936 teeth, data collected over 7 years)	97% at 8 years		
Chen 2007 (1,557,547 teeth, data collected over 1 year)	91.1%–95.4% at 5 years		
Lumley *et al.* 2008 (30,843 teeth, data collected over 10 years)	74% at 10 years	Success rate of secondary root canal treatment (Ng *et al.* 2008) Pooled weighted success from 17 studies	76.7% using 'strict' criteria (95% CI: 73.6%, 89.6%) 77.2% using 'loose' criteria (95% CI: 61.1%, 88.1%)
Tickle *et al.* 2008 (174 teeth, data collected over 5 years)	90.8% at 5 years		
Ng *et al.* 2010 (Meta-analysis of 14 studies)	86% (95% CI: 75%, 98%) at 2–3 years 93% (95% CI: 92%, 94%) at 4–5 years 87% (95% CI: 82%, 92%) at 8–10 years		
Ng *et al.* 2011b (4 year cumulative survival of 759 teeth having undergone primary root canal treatment and 858 teeth having undergone secondary root canal treatment)	95.4% (95% CI: 93.6%, 96.8%) for primary root canal treatment 95.3% (95% CI: 93.6%, 96.5%) for secondary root canal treatment	Success rate of root canal treatment (Ng *et al.* 2011a)	83% for primary root canal treatment (95% CI: 81%, 85%) 80% for secondary root canal treatment (95% CI: 78%, 82%)

and Ochi 2000a, b; Setzer and Kim 2014). In contrast, the success rate of root canal treatment provided by specialists is 98.1% compared to 89.7% for generalists at 5 years post treatment (Alley et al. 2004).

Endodontically treated teeth that have been reported to fail due to periodontal reasons have been in the region of 23–32% of cases (Chen et al. 2008; Vire 1991). Although it is possible that perio–endo lesions may have a poorer prognosis, in view of the potential outcomes of periodontal treatment and endodontic treatment, attempts to save such teeth may be beneficial. Ensuring that treatment (both endodontic and periodontal) is performed as soon as possible is important. The survival rates of teeth of poor prognosis when treated endodontically can be comparatively better than survival of implants placed in previously periodontally diseased sites (Cortellini et al. 2011, 2020; Ong et al. 2008).

References

Abbott PV. Medicaments: aids to success in endodontics. Part 1. A review of the literature. Aust Dent J. 1990a;35:438–48.

Abbott PV. Medicaments: aids to success in endodontics. Part 2. Clinical recommendations. Aust Dent J. 1990b;35:449–56.

Abbott PV. Assessing restored teeth with pulp and periapical diseases for the presence of cracks, caries and marginal breakdown. Aust Dent J. 2004;49(1):33–9.

Abbott PV, Salgado JC. Strategies for the endodontic management of concurrent endodontic and periodontal diseases. Aust Dent J. 2009;54:S70–85.

Abbott PV, Yu C. A clinical classification of the status of the pulp and the root canal system. Aust Dent J. 2007;52(1 Suppl):S17–31.

Ahmad IA. Rubber dam usage for endodontic treatment: a review. Int Endod J. 2009;42(11):963–72.

Akifusa S, Soh I, Ansai T, Hamasaki T, Takata Y, Yohida A, Fukuhara M, Sonoki K, Takehara T. Relationship of number of remaining teeth to health related quality of life in community dwelling elderly. Gerodontology. 2005;22(2):91–7.

Alghaithy RA, Qualtrough AJ. Pulp sensibility and vitality tests for diagnosing pulpal health in permanent teeth: a critical review. Int Endod J. 2017;50(2):135–42.

Alley BS, Kitchens GG, Alley L, Eleazer PD. A comparison of survival of teeth following endodontic treatment performed by general dentists or by specialists. Oral Surg Oral Med Oral Pathol Oral Radiol Endod. 2004;98(1):115–8.

Athanassiadis B, George GA, Abbott PV, Wash LJ. A review of the effects of formaldehyde release from endodontic materials. International Endodontic Journal. 2015;48:829–838.

Baba K, Igarashi Y, Nishiyama A, John MT, Akagawa Y, Ikebe K, Ishigami T. The relationship between missing occlusal units and oral health related quality of life in patients with shortened dental arches. Int J Prosthodont. 2008;21(1):72–4.

Ba-Hattab R, Al-Jamie M, Aldreib H, Alessa L, Alonazi M. Calcium hydroxide in endodontics: an overview. Open J Stomatol. 2016;6:274–89.

Bahrololoomi Z, Soleymani AA, Modaresi J, Imanian M, Lotfian M. Accuracy of an electronic apex locator for working length determination in primary anterior teeth. J Dent. 2015;12(4):243–8.

Banerji S, Mehta SB, Millar BJ. Cracked tooth syndrome. Part 1: aetiology and diagnosis. Br Dent J. 2008a;208(10):459–63.

Banerji S, Mehta SB, Millar BJ. Cracked tooth syndrome. Part 2: restorative options for the management of cracked tooth syndrome. Br Dent J. 2008b;208(11):503–14.

Baugh D, Wallace J. The role of apical instrumentation in root canal treatment: a review of the literature. J Endod. 2005;31(5):333–40.

Bender, et al. Roentgenographic and direct observation of experimental lesions in bone I & II. J Am Dent Assoc. 1961;62:152–60.

Bender IB, Seltzer S, Soltanoff W. Endodontic success – a reappraisal of criteria I. Oral Surg Oral Med Oral Pathol. 1966a;22:780–9.

Bender IB, Seltzer S, Soltanoff W. Endodontic success – a reappraisal of criteria II. Oral Surg Oral Med Oral Pathol. 1966b;22:790–802.

Bergenholtz G, Nyman S. Endodontic complications following periodontal and prosthetic treatment of patients with advanced periodontal disease. J Periodontol. 1984;55(2):63–8.

Blomlöf L, Lengheden A, Lindskog S. Endodontic infection and calcium hydroxide-treatment. Effects on periodontal healing in mature and immature replanted monkey teeth. J Clin Periodontol. 1992;19(9 Pt 1):652–8.

Bonsor SJ, Nichol R, Reid TMS, Pearson GJ. An alternative regimen for root canal disinfection. Br Dent J. 2006;201(2):101–5.

Brennan DS, Spencer AJ, Roberts-Thomson KF. Tooth loss, chewing ability and quality of life. Qual Life Res. 2008;17(2):227–35.

Bystrom A, Sundqvist G. Bacteriologic evaluation of the effect of 0.5% sodium hypochlorite in endodontic therapy. Oral Surg Oral Med Oral Pathol. 1983;5:07–12.

Calt S, Serper A. Time dependent effects of EDTA on dentine structures. J Endod. 2002;26:459–61.

Cameron CE. Cracked tooth syndrome. J Am Dent Assoc. 1964;68:405–11.

Chapple ILC, Lumley PJ. The Perio-Endo interface. Dent Update. 1999;26:331–41.

Chen E, Abbott PV. Dental pulp testing: a review. Int J Dent. 2009:365785. https://doi.org/10.1155/2009/365785. Epub 2009 Nov 12

Chen SC, Chueh LH, Hsiao CK, Tsai MY, Ho SC, Chiang CP. An epidemiologic study of tooth retention after nonsurgical endodontic treatment in a large population in Taiwan. J Endod. 2007;33(3):226–9.

Chen SC, Chueh LH, Hsiao CK, Wu HP, Chiang CP. First untoward events and reasons for tooth extraction after nonsurgical endodontic treatment in Taiwan. J Endod. 2008;34(6):671–4.

Cheung GSP. A preliminary investigation into the longevity and causes of failure of single-unit extracoronal restorations. J Dent. 1991;19:160–3.

Cheung GS. Survival of first-time nonsurgical root canal treatment performed in a dental teaching hospital. Oral Surg Oral Med Oral Pathol Oral Radiol Endod. 2002;93(5):596–604.

Cheung GSP, Lai SCN, Ng RPY. Fate of vital pulps beneath a metal ceramic crown or bridge retainer. Int Endod J. 2005;38(8):521–30.

Cheung AWT, Lee AHC, Cheung GSP. Clinical efficacy of activated irrigation in endodontics: a focused review. Restor Dent Endod. 2021;46(1):e10.

Connert T, Judenhofer MS, Hulber-J M, Schell S, Mannheim JG, Pichler BJ, Lost C, ElAyouti A. Evaluation of the accuracy of nine electronic apex locators by using micro-CT. Int Endod J. 2018;51:223–32.

Cortellini P, Stalpers G, Mollo A, Tonetti MS. Periodontal regeneration versus extraction and prosthetic replacement of teeth severely compromised by attachment loss to the apex: 5-year results of an ongoing randomized clinical trial. J Clin Periodontol. 2011;38(10):915–24.

Cortellini P, Stalpers G, Mollo A, Tonetti MS. Periodontal regeneration versus extraction and dental implant or prosthetic replacement of teeth severely compromised by attachment loss to the apex: a randomized controlled clinical trial reporting 10-year outcomes, survival analysis and mean cumulative cost of recurrence. J Clin Periodontol. 2020;47(6):768–76.

Cunningham PR, Ferguson GW. The instruction of rubber dam technique. J Am Acad Gold Foil Oper. 1970;13(1):5–12.

Dawood A, Patel S. The Dental Practicality Index – assessing the restorability of teeth. Br Dent J. 2017;222(10):755–8.

Del Fabbro M, Taschieri S, Testori T, Francetti L, Weinstein RL. Surgical versus non-surgical endodontic re- treatment for periradicular lesions. Cochrane Database Syst Rev. 2007;3:CD005511.

Doyle SL, Hodges JS, Pesun IJ, Law AS, Bowles WR. Retrospective cross sectional comparison of initial nonsurgical endodontic treatment and single-tooth implants. J Endod. 2006;32:822–7.

Doyle SL, Hodges JS, Pesun IJ, Baisden MK, Bowles WR. Factors affecting outcome of single tooth implants and endodontic restorations. J Endod. 2007;33(4):399–402.

Driscoll CO, Dowker SEP, Anderson P, Wilson RM, Gulabivala K. Effects of sodium hypochlorite on root dentine composition. J Mater Sci Mater Med. 2002;12:219–23.

Dugas NN, Lawrence HP, Teplitsky P, Friedman S. Quality of life and satisfaction outcomes of endodontic treatment. J Endod. 2002;28(12):819–27.

Eliyas S, Briggs PF, Porter RW. Antimicrobial irrigants in endodontic therapy. 2: clinical tips for isolation and irrigant use. Dent Update. 2010;37(7):463–72.

Eliyas S, Vere J, Ali Z, Harris I. Micro-surgical endodontics. Br Dent J. 2014;216(4):169–77.

Eliyas S, Jalili J, Martin N. Restoration of the root canal treated tooth. Br Dent J. 2015;218(2):53–62.

Estrela C, Estrela CRA, Barbin EL, Spano JCE, Marchesan MA, Pecora JD. Mechanism of action of sodium hypochlorite. Braz Dent J. 2002;3(2):113–7.

European Society of Endodontology. Quality guidelines for endodontic treatment: consensus report of the European Society of Endodontology. Int Endod J. 2006;39:921–30.

European Society of Endodontology (ESE) developed by: Patel S, Brown J, Semper M, Abella F, Mannocci F. European Society of Endodontology position statement: use of cone beam computed tomography in Endodontics. Int Endod J. 2019;52(12):1675–8.

Fairbourn DR, McWalter GM, Montgomery S. The effect of four preparation techniques on the amount of apically extruded debris. J Endod. 1987;13(3):102–8.

Farzaneh M, Abitbol S, Friedman S. Treatment outcome in endodontics: the Toronto study. Phases I and II: orthograde retreatment. J Endod. 2004;30(9):627–33.

Field JW, Gutmann JL, Solomon ES, Rakusin H. A clinical radiographic retrospective assessment of the success rate of single-visit root canal treatment. Int Endod J. 2004;37(1):70–82.

Figini L, Lodi G, Gorni F, Gagliani M. Single versus multiple visits for endodontic treatment of permanent teeth: a Cochrane systematic review. J Endod. 2008;34(9):1041–7.

Fox K, Youngson CC. Diagnosis and treatment of the cracked tooth. Prim Dent Care. 1997;4(3):109–13.

Friedman S. Prognosis of initial endodontic therapy. Endod Top. 2002:59–88.

Friedman S, Mor C. The success of endodontic therapy – healing and functionality. J Can Dent Assoc. 2004;32:496–503.

Gatten DL, Riedy CA, Hong SK, Johnson JD, Cohenca N. Quality of life of endodontically treated versus implant treated patients: a university-based qualitative research study. J Endod. 2011;37(7):903–9.

Gilbert GH, Meng X, Duncan RP, Shelton BJ. Incidence of tooth loss and prosthetic dental care: effect of chewing difficulty onset, a component of oral health related quality of life. J Am Geriatr Soc. 2004;52(6):880–5.

Gordon MPJ, Chandler NP. Electronic apex locators. Int Endod J. 2004;37:425–37.

Grossman LI, Oliet S. Diagnosis and treatment of endodontic emergencies. Chicago: Quintessence Publishing Co.; 1981. p. 25–6.

Haapasalo M, Endal U, Zandi H, Coli JM. Eradication of endodontic infection by instrumentation and irrigation solutions. Endod Topics. 2005;10:77–102.

Hamasha AA, Hatiwsh A. Quality of life and satisfaction of patients after nonsurgical primary root canal treatment provided by undergraduate students, graduate students and endodontic specialists. Int Endod J. 2013;46(12):1131–9.

Hannahan JP, Eleazer PD. Comparison of success of implants versus endodontically treated teeth. J Endod. 2008;34(11):1302–5.

Hargreaves KM, Cohen S, Berman LH. Cohen's pathways of the pulp. 10th ed. St. Louis: Mosby Elsevier; 2011.

Heise AL. Time required in rubber dam placement. ASDC J Dent Child. 1971;38(2):116–7.

Heling B, Heling I. Endodontic procedures must never be performed without the rubber dam. Oral Surg Oral Med Oral Pathol. 1977;43(3):464–6.

Huang Y-H, Xie S-J, Wang N-N, Ge J-Y. Status of bacterial colonization in teeth associated with different types of pulpal and periradicular disease: a scanning electron microscopy analysis. J Dent Sci. 2015;10:95e101.

Hülsmann M, Heckendorff M, Lennon A. Chelating agents in root canal treatment: mode of action and indications for their use. Int Endod J. 2003;36:810–30.

Hülsmann M, Peters OA, Dummer PMH. Mechanical preparation of root canals: shaping goals, techniques and means. Endod Top. 2005;10(1):30–76.

Hülsmann M, Rodig T, Nordmeyer S. Complications during root canal irrigation. Endo Topics. 2007;16(1):27–63.

Iqbal MK, Kim S. For teeth requiring endodontic treatment, what are the differences in outcomes of restored endodontically treated teeth compared to implant-supported restorations? Int J Oral Maxillofac Implants. 2007;22:96–116. Erratum in: Int J Oral Maxillofac Implants. 2008;23(1):56

Jena A, Sahoo SK, Govind S. Root canal irrigants: a review of their interactions, benefits, and limitations. Compend Contin Educ Dent. 2015;36(4):256–61.

Kahler W. The cracked tooth conundrum: terminology, classification, diagnosis and management. Am J Dent. 2008;21(5):275–82.

Khademi A, Yazdizadeh M, Feizianfard M. Determination of the minimum instrumentation size for penetration of irrigants to the apical third of root canal systems. J Endod. 2006;32(5):417–20.

Kim D, Kim E. Antimicrobial effect of calcium hydroxide as an intracanal medicament in root canal treatment: a literature review – Part I. In vitro studies. Restor Dent Endod. 2014;39(4):241–52. https://doi.org/10.5395/rde.2014.39.4.241.

Kim D, Kim E. Antimicrobial effect of calcium hydroxide as an intracanal medicament in root canal treatment: a literature review - Part II. in vivo studies. Restor Dent Endod. 2015;40(2):97–103.

Kim S, Kratchman S. Modern endodontic surgery concepts and practice: a review. J Endod. 2006;32(7):601–23.

Lazarski MP, Walker WA, Flores CM, Schindler WG, Hargreaves KM. Epidemiological evaluation of the outcomes of non-surgical root canal treatment in a large cohort of insured dental patients. J Endod. 2001;27:791–6.

Lengheden A, Blomlof L, Lindskog S. Effect of immediate calcium hydroxide treatment and permanent root-filling on periodontal healing in contaminated replanted teeth. Scand J Dent Res. 1991a;99:139–46.

Lengheden A, Blomlof L, Lindskog S. Effect of delayed calcium hydroxide treatment on periodontal healing in contaminated replanted teeth. Scand J Dent Res. 1991b;99:147–53.

Lin J, Chandler NP. Electric pulp testing: a review. Int Endod J. 2008;41:365–74.

Lubisich EB, Hilton TJ, Ferracane J. Cracked teeth: a review of the literature. J Esthet Restor Dent. 2010;22:158–67.

Lumley PJ, Lucarotti PS, Burke FJ. Ten-year outcome of root fillings in the General Dental Services in England and Wales. Int Endod J. 2008;41(7):577–85.

Mack F, Schwahn C, Feine JS, Mundt T, Bernhardt O, John U, Kocher PT, Biffar R. The impact of tooth loss on general health related to quality of life among elderly Pomeranians: results from the study of health in Pomerania (SHIP-O). Int J Prosthodont. 2005;18(5):414–9.

Madison S, Wilcox LR. An evaluation of coronal microleakage in endodontically treated teeth. Part III. In vivo study. J Endod. 1988;14(9):455–8.

McCabe PS, Dummer PM. Pulp canal obliteration: an endodontic diagnosis and treatment challenge. Int Endod J. 2012;45(2):177–97.

McDonald A, Setchell D. Developing a tooth restorability index. Dent Update. 2005;32:343–4.

Morris HF, Ochi S. Influence of two different approaches to reporting implant survival outcomes for five different prosthodontic applications. Ann Periodontol. 2000a;5:90–100.

Morris HF, Ochi S. Influence of research centre on overall survival outcomes at each phase of treatment. Ann Periodontol. 2000b;5:129–36.

Morris MF, Kirkpatrick TC, Rutledge RE, Schindler WG. Comparison of nonsurgical root canal treatment and single-tooth implants. J Endod. 2009;35:1325–30.

Nair PNR. On the causes of persistent apical periodontitis: a review. Int Endod J. 2006;39:249–81.

Naoum HJ, Chandler NP. Review: temporisation for endodontics. Int Endod J. 2002;35:964–78.

Ng Y-L, Mann V, Rahbaran S, Lewsey J, Gulabivala K. Outcome of primary root canal treatment: systematic review of the literature – Part 1. Effects of study characteristics on probability of success. Int Endod J. 2007;40:921–39.

Ng Y-L, Mann V, Gulabivala K. Outcome of secondary root canal treatment: a systematic review of the literature. Int Endod J. 2008;41:1026–46.

Ng Y-L, Mann V, Gulabivala K. Tooth survival following non-surgical root canal treatment: a systematic review of the literature. Int Endod J. 2010;43:171–89.

Ng YL, Mann V, Gulabivala K. A prospective study of the factors affecting outcomes of nonsurgical root canal treatment: part 1: periapical health. Int Endod J. 2011a;44(7):583–609.

Ng Y-L, Mann V, Gulabivala K. A prospective study of the factors affecting outcomes of non-surgical root canal treatment: part 2: tooth survival. Int Endod J. 2011b;44:610–25.

Niesten D, Van Mourik K, Van Der Sanden W. The impact of having natural teeth on the QoL of frail dentulous older people. A qualitative study. BMC Public Health. 2012;12:839.

Nygaard-Østby B. Chelation in root canal therapy: ethylenediaminetetraacetic acid for cleansing and widening of root canals. Odontologisk Tadskrift. 1957;65:3–11.

Oliver CM, Abbott PV. Correlation between clinical success and apical dye penetration. Int Endod J. 2001;34:637–44.

Ong CT, Ivanovski S, Needleman IG, Retzepi M, Moles DR, Tonetti MS, Donos N. Systematic review of implant outcomes in treated periodontitis subjects. J Clin Periodontol. 2008;35(5):438–62.

Paqué F, Balmer M, Attin T, Peters OA. Preparation of oval-shaped root canals in mandibular molars using nickel-titanium rotary instruments: a micro-computed tomography study. J Endod. 2010;36:703–7.

Paqué F, Zehnder M, De-Deus G. Microtomography-based comparison of reciprocating single-file F2 ProTaper technique versus rotary full sequence. J Endod. 2011;37:1394–7.

Paredes-Vieyra J, Enriquez FJ. Success rate of single- versus two-visit root canal treatment of teeth with apical periodontitis: a randomized controlled trial. J Endod. 2012;38(9):1164–9.

Patel S, Brown J, Pimentel T, Kelly RD, Abella F, Durack C. Cone beam computed tomography in endodontics – a review of the literature. Int Endod J. 2019;52(8):1138–52.

Peters DD, Baumgartner JC, Lorton L. Adult pulpal diagnosis. I. Evaluation of the positive and negative responses to cold and electrical pulp tests. J Endod. 1994;20(10):506–11.

Peters LB, Wesselink PR. Periapical healing of endodontically treated teeth in one and two visits obturated in the presence or absence of detectable microorganisms. Int Endod J. 2002;35(8):660–7.

Peters OA, Laib A, Göhring TN, Barbakow F. Changes in root canal geometry after preparation assessed by high resolution computed tomography. J Endod. 2001;27:1–6.

Petersson K, Söderström C, Kiani-Anaraki M, Lévy G. Evaluation of the ability of thermal and electrical tests to register pulp vitality. Endod Dent Traumatol. 1999;15(3):127–31.

Petersson A, Axelsson S, Davidson T, Frisk F, Hakeberg M, Kvist T, Norlund A, Mejàre I, Portenier I, Sandberg H, Tranaeus S, Bergenholtz G. Radiological diagnosis of periapical bone tissue lesions in endodontics: a systematic review. Int Endod J. 2012;45(9):783–801.

Pierce A, Lindskog S. The effect of an antibiotic / corticosteroid paste on inflammatory root resorption in vivo. Oral Surg Oral Med Oral Pathol. 1987;64:216–20.

Pierce A, Heithersay G, Lindskog S. Evidence for direct inhibition of dentinoclasts by a corticosteroid / antibiotic endodontic paste. Endod Dent Traumatol. 1988;4:44–5.

Porter RWJ, Poyser NJ, Briggs PF. A life-threatening event from poorly managed dental pain – a case report. Br Dent J. 2007;202(4):203–6.

Pratt I, Aminoshariae A, Montagnese TA, Williams KA, Khalighinejad N, Mickel A. Eight-year retrospective study of the critical time lapse between root canal completion and crown placement: its influence on the survival of endodontically treated teeth. J Endod. 2016;42(11):1598–603.

Radcliffe CE, Potouridou L, Qureshi R, Habahbeh N, Qualtrough A, Worthington H, Drucker DB. Antimicrobial activity of varying concentrations of sodium hypochlorite on the endodontic microorganisms Actinomyces isrealii, A naeslindi, Candida albicans and Enterococcus faecalis. Int Endod J. 2004;7:38–446.

Ray HA, Trope M. Periapical status of endodontically treated teeth in relation to the technical quality of the root filling and the coronal restoration. Int Endod J. 1995;28(1):12–8.

Real DG, Davidowicz H, Moura-Netto C, Zenkner Cde L, Pagliarin CM, Barletta FB, de Moura AA. Accuracy of working length determination using 3 electronic apex locators and direct digital radiography. Oral Surg Oral Med Oral Pathol Oral Radiol Endod. 2011;111(3):e44–9.

Reuter JE. The isolation of teeth and the protection of patient during endodontic treatment. Int Endod J. 1983;16(4):173–81.

Ricucci D. Apical limit of root canal instrumentation and obturation, part 1. Literature review. Int Endod J. 1998;31(6):384–93.

Ricucci D, Langeland K. Apical limit of root canal instrumentation and obturation, part 2. A histological study. Int Endod J. 1998;31(6):394–409.

Rotstein I, Simon JH. Diagnosis, prognosis and decision-making in the treatment of combined periodontal-endodontic lesions. Periodontol. 2004;34:165–203.

Salehrabi R, Rotstein I. Endodontic treatment outcomes in a large patient population in the USA: an epidemiological study. J Endod. 2004;30(12):846–50.

Salgar AR, Singh SH, Podar RS, Kulkarni GP, Babel SN. Determining predictability and accuracy of thermal and electrical dental pulp tests: an in vivo study. J Conserv Dent. 2017;20:46–9.

Saunders WP, Saunders EM. Coronal leakage as a cause of failure in root canal therapy: a review. Endod Dent Traumatol. 1994;10(3):105–8.

Saunders WP, Saunders EM. Prevalence of periradicular periodontitis associated with crowned teeth in an adult Scottish subpopulation. Br Dent J. 1998;185(3):137–40.

Schilder H. Cleaning and shaping the root canal. Dent Clin N Am. 1974;18:269–96.

Seidberg B, Schilder H. An evaluation of EDTA in endodontics. Oral Surg Oral Med Oral Pathol. 1974;37:609–20.

Seltzer S, Bender IB, Ziontz M. The dynamics of pulp inflammation: correlations between diagnostic data and actual histologic findings in the pulp. Oral Surg Oral Med Oral Pathol. 1963;16:969–77.

Setzer FC, Kim S. Comparison of long-term survival of implants and endodontically treated teeth. J Dent Res. 2014;93(1):19–26.

Shacham M, Levin A, Shemesh A, Lvovsky L, Itzhak JB, Solomonov M. Accuracy and stability of electronic apex locator length measurements in root canals with wide apical foramen: an ex vivo study. BDJ Open. 2020;202(6):22.

Shovelton DS. The presence and distribution of microorganisms within non-vital teeth. Br Dent J. 1964;117:101–7.

Silva RF, Martins EC, Prado FB, Júnior JR, Júnior ED. Endoscopic removal of an endodontic file accidentally swallowed: clinical and legal approaches. Aust Endod J. 2011;37(2):76–8.

Silveira LF, Martos J, Pintado LS, Teixeira RA, César Neto JB. Early flaring and crown-down shaping influences the first file bind to the canal apical third. Oral Surg Oral Med Oral Pathol Oral Radiol Endod. 2008;106(2):e99–101.

Silveira LF, Silveira CF, Castro LA, César Neto JB, Martos J. Crown-down preflaring in the determination of the first apical file. Braz Oral Res. 2010;24(2):153–7.

Simon JH, Glick DH, Frank AL. The relationship of endodontic-periodontic lesions. J Periodontol. 1972;43:202–8.

Singh S, Garg A. Incidence of post-operative pain after single visit and multiple visit root canal treatment: a randomized controlled trial. J Conserv Dent. 2012;15(4):323–7.

Sirtes G, Waltimo T, Schaetzle M, Zehnder. The effect of temperature on sodium hypochlorite: short term stability, pulp dissolution capacity and antimicrobial efficacy. J Endod. 2005;1(9):669–71.

Sjogren U, Hagglund B, Sundqvist G, Wing K. Factors affecting the long-term results of endodontic treatment. J Endod. 1990;16:498–504.

Solomon C, Chalfin H, Kellert M, Weseley P. The endodontic-periodontal lesion: a rational approach to treatment. J Am Dent Assoc. 1995;126(4):473–9.

Spangberg L, Engstrom B, Langeland K. Biological effect of dental materials. 3. toxicity and antimicrobial effect of endodontic antiseptics in vitro. Oral Surg Oral Med Oral Pathol. 1973;36(6):856–71.

Stewardson DA, McHugh ES. Patients' attitudes to rubber dam. Int Endod J. 2002;35(10):812–9.

Strindberg LZ. The dependence of the results of pulp therapy on certain factors. An analytic study based on radio-graphic and clinical follow-up examinations. Acta Odontol Scand. 1956;14(Suppl. 21):1–175.

Teixeira CS, Felippe MC, Felippe W. The effect of application time of EDTA and NaOCl on intracanal smear layer removal: an SEM analysis. Int Endod J. 2005;38(5):285–90.

Tickle M, Milsom K, Qualtrough A, Blinkhorn F, Aggarwal VR. The failure rate of NHS funded molar endodontic treatment delivered in general dental practice. Br Dent J. 2008;204(5):E8; discussion 254–5

Tomson R, Polycarpou N, Tomson P. Contemporary obturation of the root canal system. Br Dent J. 2014;216:315–22.

Torabinejad M, Ung B, Kettering JD. In vitro bacterial penetration of coronally unsealed endodontically treated teeth. J Endod. 1990;16:566–9.

Torabinejad M, Anderson P, Bader J, Brown LJ, Chen LH, Goodacre CJ, Kattadiyil MT, Kutsenko D, Lozada J, Patel R, Petersen F, Puterman I, White SN. Outcomes of root canal treatment and restoration, implant-supported single crowns, fixed partial dentures, and extraction without replacement: a systematic review. J Prosthet Dent. 2007;98(4):285–311.

Tronstad L, Barnett F, Riso K, Slots L. Extraradicular endodontic infections. Endod Dent Traumatol. 1987;3:86–90.

Tronstad L, Barnett F, Cervone F. Periapical bacterial plaque in teeth refractory to endodontic treatment. Endod Dent Traumatol. 1990;6:73–7.

Tsesis I, Rosen E, Taschieri S, Telishevsky Strauss Y, Ceresoli V, Del Fabbro M. Outcomes of surgical endodontic treatment performed by a modern technique: an updated meta-analysis of the literature. J Endod. 2013;39(3):332–9.

Uzunoglu-Özyürek E, Karaaslan H, Türker SA, Özçelik B. Influence of size and insertion depth of irrigation needle on debris extrusion and sealer penetration. Restor Dent Endod. 2017;43(1):e2.

Van Nieuwenhuysen JP, Aouar M, D'Hoore W. Retreatment or radiographic monitoring in endodontics. Int Endod J. 1994;27(2):75–81.

Vernillo AT, Ramamurthy NS, Golub LN, Rifkin BR. The non-antimicrobial properties of tetracycline for the treatment of periodontal disease. Curr Opin Periodontol. 1994;2:111–8.

Vire DE. Failure of endodontically treated teeth: classification and evaluation. J Endod. 1991;17(7):338–42.

von Arx T, Jensen SS, Janner SFM, Hänni S, Bornstein MM. A 10-year follow-up study of 119 teeth treated with apical surgery and root-end filling with mineral trioxide aggregate. J Endod. 2019;45(4):394–401.

Weiger R, Rosendahl R, Lost C. Influence of calcium hydroxide intracanal dressings on the prognosis of teeth with endodontically induced periapical lesions. Int Endod J. 2000;33(3):219–26.

Weinreb MM, Meier E. The relative efficiency of EDTA, sulfuric acid and mechanical instrumentation in the enlargement of root canals. Oral Surg Oral Med Oral Pathol. 1965;19:247–52.

Wolfart S, Heydecke G, Luthardt RG, Marre B, Freesmeyer WB, Stark H, et al. Effects of prosthetic treatment for shortened dental arches on oral health-related quality of life, self-reports of pain and jaw disability: results from the pilot-phase of a randomized multicentre trial. J Oral Rehabil. 2005;32:815–22.

Yared GM, Dagher FE. Influence of apical enlargement on bacterial infection during treatment of apical periodontitis. J Endod. 1994;20:535–7.

Young GR, Parashos P, Messer HH. The principles of techniques for cleaning root canals. Aust Dent J Suppl. 2007;52(1 Suppl):S52–63.

Zehnder M. Root canal irrigants. J Endod. 2006;32(5):389–98.

Zehnder M, Gold SI, Hasselgren G. Pathologic interaction in pulpal and periodontal tissues. J Clin Periodontol. 2002;29:663–71.

Abstract

The previous chapters have discussed isolated periodontal and endodontic lesions, their diagnosis, management and the outcomes of treatment. The following chapter considers the two disease processes together, and discusses the classification of Perio-Endo lesions.

Perio-Endo Lesions

The endodontic lesion occurs after pulpal necrosis as a result of pulpal exposure to microbes (via caries, cracks, trauma), and may present with a sinus tract to establish drainage, however, should heal within 3–6 months of endodontic treatment (Simon et al. 1972). This is a primary endodontic lesion. It may then develop a secondary periodontal component if plaque accumulation in the sinus tract, leading to breakdown of the periodontal ligament and downgrowth of the epithelium, requiring both endodontic and periodontal treatment (Gargiulo 1984). The periodontal lesion occurs as a result of a combination of infection and inflammation, leading to the destruction of the gingival connective tissue, periodontal ligament and alveolar bone, with possible denuding of the cemental layer and resorption. The endotoxins created prevent repair (Kenkins and Allan 1994). In a primary periodontal lesion, although the bone loss may have reached the apex of the root, the pulp tissue remains vital, requiring only non-surgical or surgical periodontal treatment. However, there can be secondary endodontic involvement if the periodontal pathogens reach the apical foramen, then periodontal disease has caused pulpal necrosis, requiring endodontic treatment as well. Table 6.1 summarises the key points.

Perio-Endo lesions are those that have a periodontal and endodontic component, with or without communication between the two (Abbott and Salgado 2009;

S. Eliyas, *The Periodontic-Endodontic Interface*, https://doi.org/10.1007/978-3-031-49937-1_6

Table 6.1 Summary of the signs and symptoms of periodontal and endodontic disease

		Endodontic lesions	Periodontal lesions
Clinical findings	Aetiology	Pulp infection	Periodontal infection
	Vitality	Non-vital	Vital
	Restorative status	Deep/extensive restoration	Not related
	Plaque/Calculus	Not related	Primary cause
	Inflammation	Acute	Chronic
	Pockets	Single/narrow pocket	Multiple, wide coronally
	pH value	Often acidic	Usually alkaline
	Trauma	Primary or secondary	Contributing factor
	Microbial status	Few microbes	Complex microbes
Radiographic findings	Pattern	Localised	Generalised (other sites)
	Periapical	Radiolucent	Not often related
	Bone loss	Wide apically	Wider coronally
	Vertical bone loss	No/sometimes	Yes/sometimes
Histopathology	Junctional epithelium	No apical migration	Apical migration
	Granulation tissue	Apical (minimum)	Coronal (larger)
	Gingivae	Normal	Some recession/inflammation
Treatment		Root canal treatment	Periodontal treatment

Kenkins and Allan 1994; Papapanou et al. 2018), however, it is not always possible to state whether the lesion originated from the periodontium or endodontium. The microbial flora can be the similar in both periodontal and endodontic infections, and if either disease is left untreated, progression can occur to the other tissue (Case 12), with also the possibility of 'cross-seeding' of bacteria from one tissue to the other in either direction (Abbot and Salgado 2009).

Classification of Perio-Endo Lesions

There are numerous proposed classifications for perio-endo lesions (Table 6.2). Most trying to identify a primary cause and secondary involvement, which is often not possible as there may be delayed presentation, with both lesions manifesting at the same time. If there are consecutive radiographs showing the development of the lesion, using such classifications may be possible.

Table 6.2 The various classifications of perio-endo lesions

Authors	Classification of Perio-Endo Lesions
Abbott and Salgado 2009	Class 1 — Concurrent endodontic and periodontal diseases without communication (infected root canal system with apical periodontitis as well as marginal periodontal breakdown, without the periodontal pocket extending to the apical lesion clinically or radiographically) Class 2 — Concurrent endodontic and periodontal diseases with communication (infected root canal system with apical periodontitis as well as marginal periodontal breakdown, with the periodontal pocket extending to the apical lesion clinically and radiographically) Class 1 may progress to Class 2 if left untreated
Rotstein & Simon 2006	1. Retrograde periodontal disease: a. Primary endodontic lesion with drainage through the PDL, b. Primary endodontic lesion with secondary periodontal involvement 2. Primary periodontal lesion 3. Primary periodontal lesion with secondary endodontic involvement 4. Combined endodontic-periodontal lesion 5. Iatrogenic periodontal lesions: a. root perforations, b. coronal leakage, c. dental injuries or trauma d. chemicals used in dentistry, c. vertical root fractures
Kim & Kratchman 2006	Class A — Absence of periradicular lesion, no mobility, normal pocket depth, but symptoms remain after non-surgical therapies have been exhausted Class B — Presence of a small periradicular lesion in the apical quarter, clinical symptoms such as discomfort/sensitivity to percussion sinus, tracts, normal periodontal probing depths, and no mobility Class C — Large periradicular lesions progressing coronally, without periodontal pockets and/or mobility Class D — clinically similar to those in Class C with periodontal pockets >4 mm and no communication of the pocket and the endodontic lesion Class E — Deep periradicular lesions with endodontic-periodontal communication to the apex, no obvious fracture Class F — Apical lesion and complete denudement of the buccal plate, no mobility

Rotstein and Simon 2004 (based on primary and secondary involvement)	Class I: Primary endodontic disease
	
	Class II: Primary periodontal disease
	
	Class III: Combined diseases, which include:
	
	  A — Primary endodontic disease with secondary periodontal involvement
	
	  B — Primary periodontal disease with secondary endodontic involvement
	
	  C — True combined diseases.

Weine 2004 (based on treatment needs)	Class I: Tooth in which symptoms clinically and radiographically simulate periodontal disease but are in fact due to pulpal inflammation and/or necrosis Class II: Tooth that has both pulpal or periapical disease and periodontal disease concomitantly Class III: Tooth has no pulpal problem but requires endodontic therapy plus root amputation to gain periodontal healing Class IV: Tooth that clinically and radiographically simulates pulpal or periapical disease but in fact has periodontal disease
Walker 2001	1. Endodontic lesions (inflammation in the periodontal tissues due to noxious agents present in the canal system). 2. Periodontal lesions (inflammation inpulpal tissues due to accumulation of plaque on the external root surface). 3. True-combined lesions (endodontic and periodontal lesions developing independently, progressing concurrently and merge at a point along the root surface). 4. Iatrogenic lesions (lesions produced as a result of treatment).
Von Arx and Cochran 2001	Class I: Perio-endo lesion with bone defect in the apex which may invade the buccal/labial and lingual cortex

(continued)

Table 6.2 (continued)

(based on treatment need)	Class II: Perio-endo lesion with an apical lesion andconcomitant marginal involvement Class III: Perio-endo lesion with a furcation lesion coming from accessory canals or from iatrogenic perforation with or without marginal involvement
Armitage 1999	1. Endodontic-periodontal lesions 2. Periodontal-endodontic lesions 3. Combined lesions
Torabinejad and Trope 1996 (based on primary and secondary involvement)	Class 1 — Periodontal defect of endodontic origin Class 2 — Periodontal defect of periodontal origin Class 3 — Combined endodontic-periodontal lesion Class 4 — Separate endodontic and periodontal lesions Class 5 — Combined lesions with communication Class 6 — Combined lesions without communication
Grossman 1981 (based on treatment needs)	1. Teeth requiring endodontic therapy alone 2. Teeth requiring periodontal therapy alone 3. Teeth requiring endodontic and periodontal therapy
Geurtsen et al 1985 (based on treatment needs)	1 — Combined lesions requiring only a single root-canal treatment (favourable prognosis) 2 — Combined lesions requiring both endodontic and periodontal treatments (less favourable prognosis) 3 — Combined lesions with little hope of successful treatment (poor prognosis)

Guldener 1985 (based on causes, primary and secondary involvement and treatment needs)	Class I: Primary endodontic lesions
	
	  a: Accidental perforations (intra-alveolar) or resorptive perforations (internal resorption)
	
	  b: Chronic periradicular lesion (granuloma or cyst) or acute periradicular lesion (alveolar abscess)
	
	Class II: Primary periodontal lesions
	
	  a: Advanced periodontal disease with or without extension to the apical area (pulp vital)
	
	  b: Secondary endodontic involvement with infection through lateral canals or dentinal tubules, and pulpal necrosis with or without secondary periapical involvement
	
	Class III: combined lesion- true combined lesion (coalescence between periodontal and endodontic lesion) or vertical crown-root fracture with pulpal involvement

Hiatt 1977 (based on primary and secondary involvement)	Class 1: Pulpal lesions with secondary periodontal disease of short duration Class 2: Pulpal lesions with secondary periodontal disease of long duration Class 3: Periodontal lesions of short duration with secondary pulpal disease Class 4: Periodontal lesions of long duration with secondary pulpal disease Class 5: Periodontal lesions treated by hemi-section or root amputation Class 6: Complete and incomplete crown-root fractures Class 7: Independent pulpal and periodontal lesions merge into a combined lesion Class 8: Pulpal lesions evolving into periodontal lesions following treatment Class 9: Periodontal lesions evolving into pulpal lesions following treatment
Simon et al 1972 (based on primary and secondary involvement)	Class I: Primary endodontic lesion (sinus tract has formed to establish drainage) Class II: Primary periodontal lesion (periodontal disease progressed to involve the apex with the tooth remaining vital) Class III: Primary endodontic disease with secondary periodontal involvement (plaque formation within the sinus tract progressing to periodontal disease) Class IV: Primary periodontal disease with secondary endodontic involvement (periodontal disease progressed to the apex of the tooth causing pulpal necrosis) Class V: True combined perio-endo lesion
Oliet and Pollock 1968 (based on primary and secondary involvement)	Class I: Primary endodontic involvement with secondary periodontal factors, requiring only endodontic treatment Class II: Primary periodontal involvement with secondary endodontic factors, requiring periodontal treatment alone Class III: Endodontic-periodontal involvement requiring correlated and combined therapy

A new classification for periodontal and peri-implant diseases was introduced in 2017 and within this, is a classification for endodontic-periodontal lesions (Jepsen 2020; Papapanou et al. 2018; Herrera et al. 2018):

1. Endo-Perio lesions with root damage (root fracture or cracking, root canal or pulp chamber perforations, external root resorption)
2. Endo-Perio lesions without root damage
    (a) Endo-perio lesions in periodontitis patients
        i. Grade 1: a deep and narrow periodontal pocket in one tooth surface
        ii. Grade 2: a deep and wide periodontal pocket in one tooth surface
        iii. Grade 3: deep pockets in more than one tooth surface
    (b) Endo-perio lesions in non-periodontitis patients
        i. Grade 1: a deep and narrow periodontal pocket in one tooth surface
        ii. Grade 2: a deep and wide periodontal pocket in one tooth surface
        iii. Grade 3: deep pockets in more than one tooth surface

The review did not find a distinct difference between the pathophysiology of an endo-perio lesion and a periodontal lesion (Papapanou et al. 2018).

Many have suggested that the origin of the infection is irrelevant to the treatment and have favoured the classifications that focus on the present state of the tooth and not the primary and secondary causes (Chapple and Lumley 1999; Abbott and Salgado 2009) as seen in Table 6.3.

The following radiographs (Figs. 6.1 and 6.2) depict apical periodontitis and marginal periodontal breakdown, with bone between the two lesions (Abbott and Salgado Class 1):

Apical periodontitis and marginal periodontal breakdown without bone between the two lesions is shown in Fig. 6.3 (Abbott and Salgado Class 2):

Table 6.3 A simplified classification of perio-endo lesions (Abbott and Salgado 2009)

Endodontic lesion	If tooth has irreversible pulpitis or is necrotic — needs endodontic treatment
Periodontal lesion	If tooth is vital with a periodontal lesion that is progressing — needs periodontal treatment
Concomitant lesions — both endodontic and periodontal lesions exist but appear not to be communicating (Class 1) **Combined lesion** — both endodontic and periodontal lesions exist and are communicating (Class 2)	Identifying the primary source of infection is irrelevant in the management if tooth is necrotic with a periodontal lesion — needs endodontic and periodontal treatment

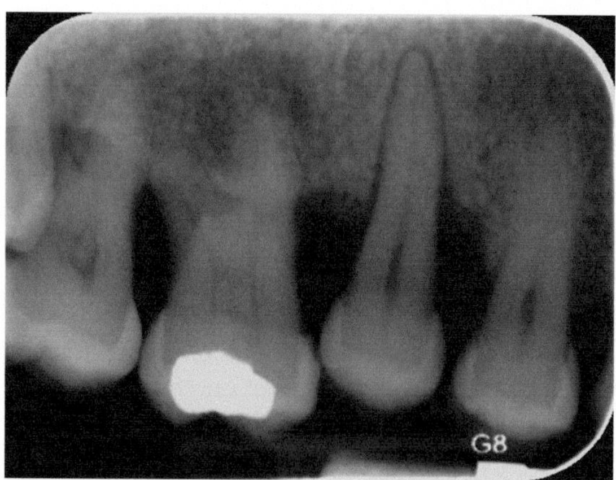

Fig. 6.1 LCPA radiograph of the UR56: There is generalised periodontal disease as can be seen by horizontal bone loss of 60–70%, with an apical radiolucency associated with the UR6. It is plausible that the UR6 has lost vitality as it is restored with an amalgam restoration that appears to be close to or even impinge on the pulp horns. The UR6 may give a positive response to electric pulp testing, as it is a multi-rooted tooth, and may have a furcation involvement or periodontal pocket. However, there appears to be bone present between the apical area and the marginal periodontal breakdown, therefore, one should expect healing of the apical area following endodontic treatment

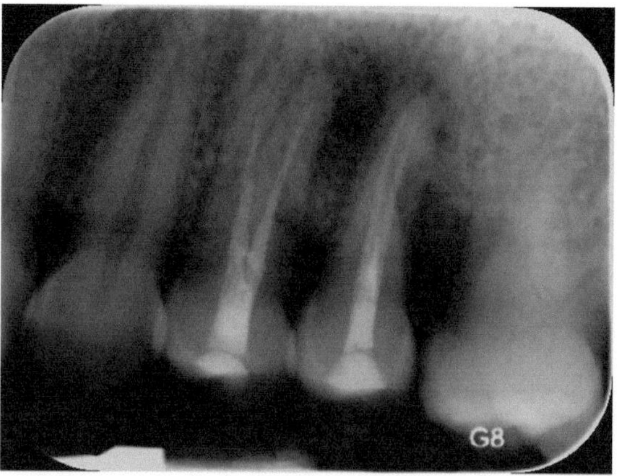

Fig. 6.2 LCPA radiograph of the UL45: There is mild generalised periodontal disease as can be seen by horizontal bone loss of 10–40%, with apical radiolucencies associated with the UL4 and UL5. It is unlikely that the apical area associated with the UL4 will be communicating with the marginal periodontal breakdown, however, the apical area associated with the UL5 may be communicating with the marginal periodontal bone loss on the distal aspect of the root. Endodontic re-treatment and periodontal treatment is likely to be required for the UL5

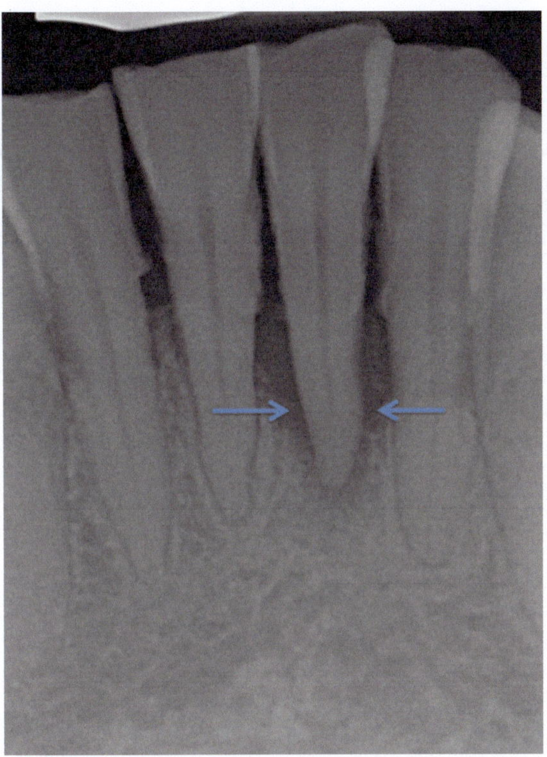

Fig. 6.3 LCPA radiograph of the lower central incisors: There is clearly periodontal disease, with 50–60% bone loss associated with the LR21, LL2 and 80% bone loss associated with the LL1 (associated with which there is also an apical widening of the periodontal ligament). Did the periodontal disease cause the apical area or is there a possibility of occlusal trauma leading to fremitus and a widened periodontal ligament? Or trauma that lead to loss of vitality and apical pathology, which now communicates with the periodontal lesion? In this type of case a thorough history, clinical examination and sensibility testing is required. In this case, once root canal treatment has been completed, only bone regeneration to the levels indicated by the arrows can be expected. Can you describe the clinical findings you expect from the LL1 and how that might inform your treatment plan?

Case 12 In some cases it is possible to further classify the lesions, beyond just the presence of a perio-endo lesion. The following radiographs (Fig. 6.4a–c) show the presence of generalised periodontal disease with vertical bone loss and apical pathology associated with teeth that are minimally or not restored. The aetiology is likely to be primary periodontal disease and secondary endodontic involvement in a non-parafunctional, fit and well patient.

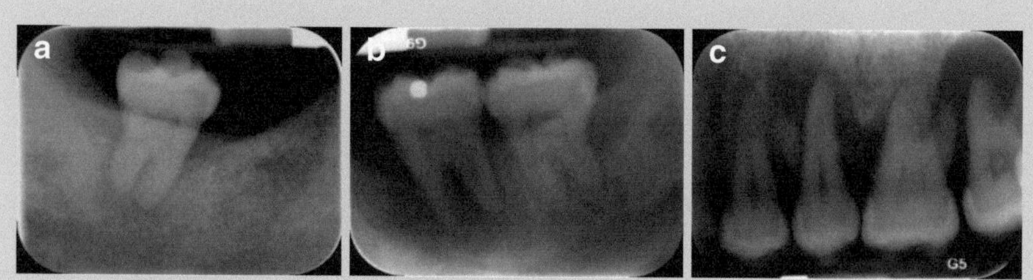

Fig 6.4 LCPA radiograph of the lower right second molar (**a**), lower left second and third molars (**b**), and UL4567 (**c**), which are all minimally restored or unrestored teeth with associated vertical bone defects and apical radiolucencies

References

Abbott PV, Salgado JC. Strategies for the endodontic management of concurrent endodontic and periodontal diseases. Aust Dent J. 2009;54:S70–85.

Armitage GC. Development of a classification system for periodontal diseases and conditions. Ann Periodontol. 1999;4:1–6.

Chapple ILC, Lumley PJ. The perio-endo interface. Dent Update. 1999;26:331–41.

Gargiulo A Jr. Endoodntic-periodontic interrelationships. Diagnosis and treatment. Dent Clin N Am. 1984;28(4):767–81.

Geurtsen W, Ehrmann EH, Löst C. Die kombinierte endodontal-parodontale Erkrankung. Deutsche Zahnärztliche Zeitschrift. 1985;40:817–22.

Grossman LI, Oliet S. Diagnosis and treatment of endodontic emergencies. Chicago: Quintessence Publishing Co.; 1981. p. 25–6.

Guldener PH. The relationship between periodontal and pulpal disease. Int Endod J. 1985;18:41–54.

Herrera D, Retamal-Valdes B, Alonso B, Feres M. Acute periodontal lesions (periodontal abscesses and necrotizing periodontal diseases) and endo-periodontal lesions. J Periodontol. 2018;89(Suppl 1):S85–S102.

Hiatt WH. Pulpal periodontal disease. J Periodontol. 1977;48:598–609.

Jepsen S. New classification of periodontal and peri-implant diseases and conditions. Endodontic Pract Today. 2020;14(1)

Kenkins WM, Allan CJ. Guide to periodontics. 3rd ed. California: Wright Publishing Company; 1994. p. P146–52.

Kim S, Kratchman S. Modern endodontic surgery concepts and practice: a review. J Endod. 2006;32(7):601–23.

Oliet S, Pollock S. Classification and treatment of endo-perio involved teeth. Bull Phila Cty Dent Soc. 1968;34:12–6.

Papapanou PN, Sanz M, Buduneli N, et al. Periodontitis: consensus report of workgroup 2 of the 2017 World workshop on the classification of periodontal and peri-implant diseases and conditions. J Periodontol. 2018;89(Suppl 1):S173–82.

Rotstein I, Simon JH. Diagnosis, prognosis and decision-making in the treatment of combined periodontal-endodontic lesions. Periodontol. 2004;34:165–203.

Rotstein I, Simon JH. The endo-perio lesion: a critical appraisal of the disease condition. Endod Topics. 2006;13:34–56.

Simon JH, Glick DH, Frank AL. The relationship of endodontic-periodontic lesions. J Periodontol. 1972;43:202–8.

Torabinejad M, Trope M. Endodontic and periodontal interrelationships. In: Walton RE, Torabinejad M, editors. Principles and practice of endodontics, vol. 4; 1996. p. 94–106.

von Arx T, Cochran DL. Rationale for the application of the GTR principle using a barrier membrane in endodontic surgery: a proposal of classification and literature review. Int J Periodontics Restorative Dent. 2001;21(127–39):9.

Walker M. The pathogenesis and treatment of endo-perio lesions. Pathogenesis. 2001;2(3):91–5.

Weine FS. Endodontic-periodontal problems. In: Weine FS, editor. Endodontic therapy. 6th ed. St. Louis: Mosby; 2004. p. 452–81.

Periodontal Infections That May Have Endodontic Manifestations

7

Abstract

This chapter describes primary periodontal lesions that may develop endodontic manifestations and present as 'perio-endo' lesions. Periodontal lesions develop as a result of a host response to microbial accumulation around the gingival tissues, resulting in inflammation and inflammatory mediators that give rise to destruction of the gingival connective tissue, periodontal ligament, alveolar bone and loss of the outer cementoblast layer.

Periodontal Lesions with Endodontic Manifestations

An intact layer of cementum is required to protect the pulp from the pathogenic byproducts of microbes within plaque (Lindhe et al. 2008). As described earlier, pulpal inflammation, secondary dentine formation and internal resorption have been associated with periodontal disease. Pulp changes have only been recorded if the periodontal pocket is deep enough to involve a large lateral canal or if the dentinal tubules are exposed as a result of denuded cementum, and the periodontal lesions extends to exposed dentinal tubules (Abbott and Salgado 2009). Even when the cementum is denuded, the pulp is protected from bacterial ingress by the outflow of dentinal fluid (Seltzer and Bender 1959; Zehnder et al. 2002). While the pulp is vital, the host response, often via fluid within the dentinal tubules, prevents the ingress of toxins and microbes into the canal system (Chapple and Lumley 1999). Although the insult of periodontal disease on the pulp has been shown to be cumulative, a periodontal pocket is unlikely to cause necrosis of the tooth until it reaches the apex of the root, with complete pulp necrosis only occurring if the periodontal pocket not only extends to the main apical foramen, but the foramen is also invaded by plaque (Langeland et al. 1974; Bergenholtz and Lindhe 1978). Once this happens, the pulpal blood supply is affected, the pulp becomes necrotic, and apical periodontitis is inevitable as microbial invasion of the canal space occurs without the vital pulpal tissue to resist bacterial invasion from the periodontal pocket. Although some studies have suggested that pulpal necrosis is possible when periodontal disease reaches accessory canals, other studies have shown that teeth with periodontal involvement can still have relatively normal pulps regardless of the severity of the periodontal disease (Zehnder et al. 2002). It is possible for teeth to have a small periapical radiolucent area seen radiographically, while still remaining vital (Langeland 1987). As long as the blood supply from the apical foramen is maintained, the pulp can withstand insult from periodontal disease. Figure 7.1 shows the various ways in which periodontal disease can lead to endodontic disease.

The treatment of periodontal disease can also cause pulpal inflammation (usually reversible pulpitis, i.e. short lasting sensitivity, mainly to cold, sometimes also heat and sweet foods), which resolves within a matter of weeks, with occasional progression to irreversible pulpitis. Topical application of fluoride toothpaste, to help seal any exposed dentinal tubules, starting after root surface debridement is helpful. The way periodontal treatment is provided will influence pulpal reactions for example scaling and root planing or administration of medicaments. Cementum acts as a protective layer from toxic products of plaque microbiota, and in the absence of numerous/large lateral canals, the cementum must be damaged and dentinal tubules

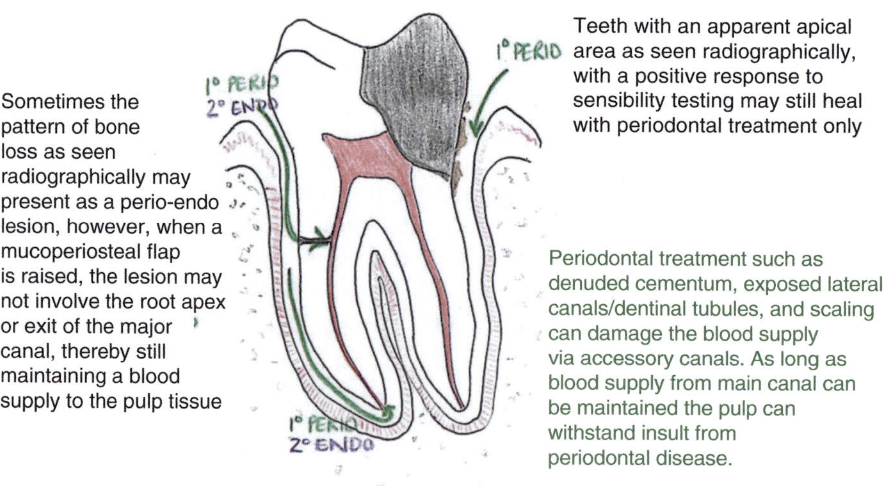

Fig. 7.1 Primary periodontal lesions leading to endodontic involvement and therefore, secondary endodontic manifestations

exposed before pulp irritation occurs. During periodontal treatment, cementum may be damaged or removed, and the blood supply via accessory canals may be damaged (Fig. 7.2). Based on the extent of root planing, there may be varying degrees of pulp inflammation depending on the amount of cementum removed, the extent to which the exposed dentine is protected by a smear layer, and the general health of the pulp (Abbott and Salgado 2009). The pulp may form various amounts of mineralisation leading to narrower canals (which may be a reparative and protective process rather than an inflammatory process), or develop fibrosis, or lead to pulpal necrosis.

Primary periodontal lesions may present as a mobile tooth with a wide/broad based pocket, with the tooth exhibiting a positive response to sensibility testing. The patient may only present with pain when the pulp becomes involved. Treatment depends on the extent of the periodontal destruction and the prognosis depends entirely on the outcome of the periodontal treatment (which in turn is very much dependent on the patient's motivation and compliance). Primary periodontal lesions that lead to secondary endodontic involvement (perio-endo lesions) may only be different from endo-perio lesions in the order of their development. They are likely to look the same clinically and radiographically when the tooth is examined in isolation, therefore, look carefully at the periodontal susceptibility generally and past periodontal treatment for each patient. The prognosis depends on the continuing periodontal treatment and subsequent endodontic treatment. The prognosis may be

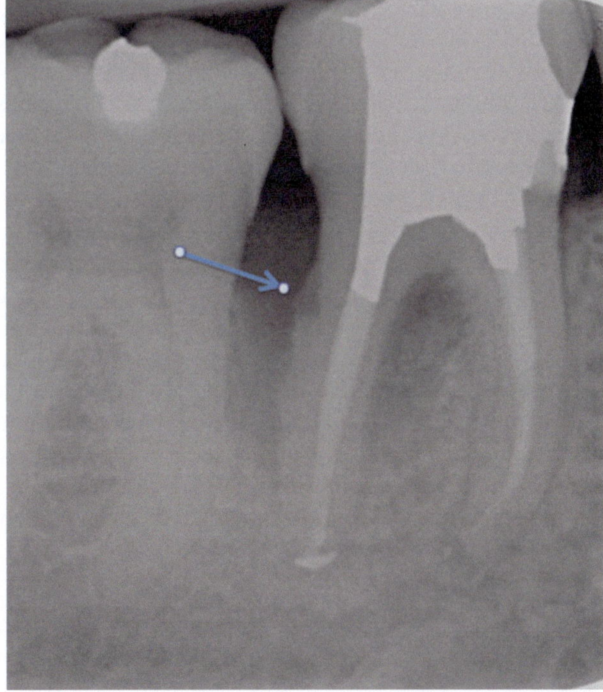

Fig. 7.2 LCPA radiograph of the LR6: Periodontal treatment can damage the cementum and root structure, especially where overzealous use of instrumentation can result in notching along the root surface as seen radiographically (arrow). When ultrasonic instrumentation is used in periodontal treatment, the tip of the ultrasonic should be kept constantly moving, in a zig-zag motion, and with light pressure. As this tooth was already heavily restored, it is difficult to assume that the periodontal treatment was the reason for the tooth losing vitality and requiring root canal treatment

poorer for single rooted teeth. In periodontal health, a palato-gingival groove is rare instant when the periodontal component causes an endodontic lesion as a result of developing a self-sustaining pocketing due to loss of attachment along the groove to reach the root apex (Kogon 1986; Lara et al. 2000; Al-Hezaimi et al. 2009; Withers et al. 1981). Occlusal trauma can lead to widening of the periodontal ligament and vertical bone loss as seen radiographically resembling periodontal disease with endodontic involvement. A periodontal pocket may mimic an apical periodontitis lesion if the pocket extends into the bone buccally or lingually/palatally, and apical to the level of the root apex, thereby being superimposed on the apex as the x-ray beam travels through it (Abbott and Salgado 2009). In these cases the apex is not involved in the lesion. Special tests to identify the status of the pulp and possible reasons for losing vitality must be considered in conjunction with radiographic findings to diagnose if an endodontic issue is present. If none can be identified, a periodontal lesion mimicking apical periodontitis must be deliberated, and reviewed after periodontal treatment.

The (Lateral) Periodontal Abscess

Periodontal disease can also require drainage through the gingival sulcus to prevent acute episodes, although, periodontal abscesses can occur in periodontally susceptible and non-susceptible individuals. When acute episodes do occur, they may present as (lateral) periodontal abscesses, and are a rare situation where periodontal disease causes acute pain. These abscesses occur when the opening of the periodontal pocket is blocked. In patients with periodontal disease, this may be as a result of calculus blocking vertical bone defects, change in microbiota (becoming more virulent) causing more suppuration or change in host response making drainage through the periodontal pocket more inefficient, or following periodontal treatment (scaling and leaving calculus behind, regenerative surgical techniques using membranes or scaffolds, or even when the sutures block the entrance to periodontal pockets, or due to tightening of the gingival cuff) trapping infection in the periodontal pocket. In periodontally sound patients, the occurrence of periodontal abscesses are also related to blockage of the opening of a shallow periodontal pocket with a foreign body such as calculus, food debris, tooth picks, dental materials or due to alterations in the root morphology such as developmental grooves, cemental tears, perforations, root fractures, and resorption defects (Herrera et al. 2018).

The prevalence of periodontal abscesses is thought to be up to 14% of all dental emergencies, worst in periodontal patients (27–37%), especially in those with active periodontal disease and in sites where coronal scaling was performed (Herrera et al. 2018). There may be rapid destruction of the periodontal apparatus of a tooth, if immediate management does not occur and can very rarely also lead to systemic consequences (Herrera et al. 2018). Untreated, the eventual result is the development of a periodontal pocket (Fig. 7.3) that migrates apically and accumulates

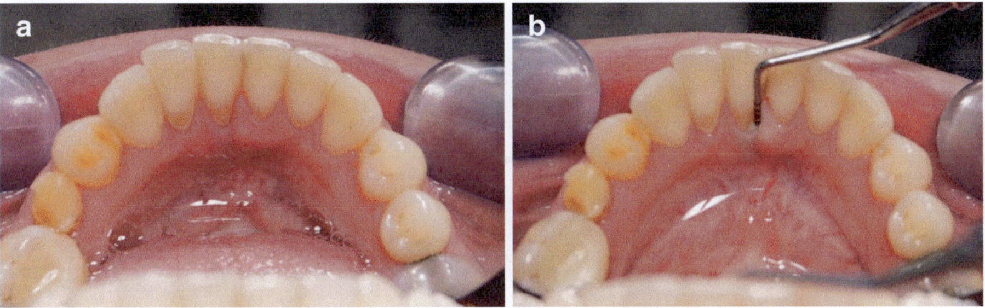

Fig. 7.3 Intra-oral photographs of the lower anterior teeth (**a** and **b**): A deep periodontal pocket of 7 mm with slight swelling of the lingual attached gingivae was seen associated with the mesial line angle on the lingual aspect of the LR1, with suppuration from the pocket (**b**). The LR1 was not tender to percussion and tested positive to sensibility testing. The gingival tissues, at first glance, appear healthy and fairly clean. Without meticulous walking of the periodontal probe, this pocket could have easily been missed. Careful visualisation of the gingival tissues does reveal thin soft tissue with a purplish appearance. The lesion may have been mistaken for an endodontic lesion, in a tooth with a potential second canal to explain the sensibility test findings. Drainage may explain the lack of tenderness to percussion, and insufficient time for the development of an apical area may explain the lack of apical pathology on a radiograph

further plaque and continues the cycle of inflammation, unless the periodontal pocket can be cleaned and the microbes disturbed daily. The management may be extraction of what is considered a 'hopeless' tooth, if repeated periodontal abscesses occur around the same tooth. The microbiology is similar to periodontal disease and histopathology reveals acute inflammatory cells in an area of necrotic connective tissue and ulcerated pocket epithelium (Herrera et al. 2018).

Clinically, lateral periodontal abscesses usually have less severe pain than a peri-radicular abscess, often with swelling before pain, and swelling and tenderness usually in the attached gingivae. The tooth usually remains vital and is not usually tender to percussion, however may be mobile. There is often an associated periodontal pocket, which may be deep, with bleeding on probing, and draining might still be through the periodontal pocket rather than a separate draining sinus. On rare occasions signs of systemic spread (temperature, malaise, facial swelling) may be evident. Radiographically, there may be marginal bone loss and a vertical bone defect (Fig. 7.4). In contrast, an acute peri-radicular abscess (as a result of endodontic disease) causes severe pain (pain may occur before the swelling, with previous symptoms of pulpitis), as well as swelling and tenderness over the apex of the causative tooth. The tooth is usually not vital (although could be partially vital) and is often very tender to percussion. Radiographically, it may be possible to see a widened periodontal ligament or apical radiolucency. The treatment of lateral periodontal abscesses is non-surgical periodontal treatment, oral hygiene instructions and supportive periodontal care.

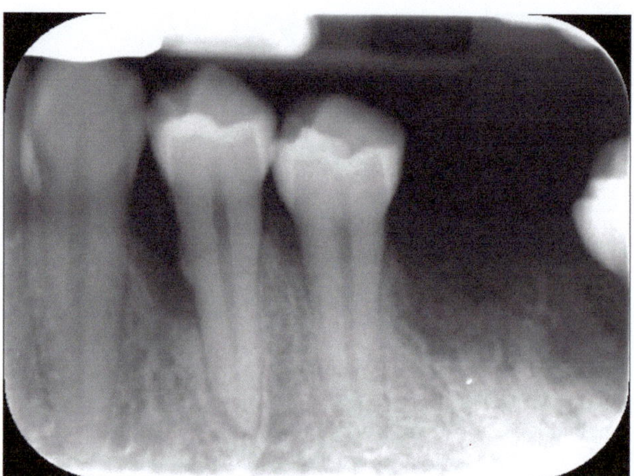

Fig. 7.4 LCPA radiograph of the LL45: Radiographic appearance of lateral periodontal abscesses, if in the right position to be seen clearly with plain film radiographs, will have this appearance. It may be possible to identify the cause. On this LL4, it is a significant amount of calculus on the mesial aspect of the root. This patient is clearly periodontally susceptible, and the presence of a plaque retentive factor, in this case porous calculus, will house a complex biofilm of periodontal pathogens, which can lead to acute exacerbation of such lesions

Epulis

Fibrous epulis often occur in the attached gingivae, and in response to chronic gingival irritation such as subgingival caries, restorations with poor subgingival margins, calculus and loss of vitality (Fonseca et al. 2014). Surgical removal of an epulis without managing the chronic irritation is likely to result in recurrence (Fig. 7.5).

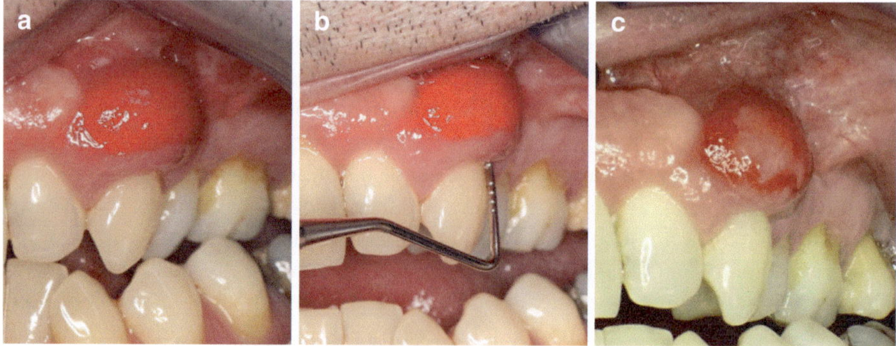

Fig. 7.5 Intra-oral photographs of the UL3: A 47-year old presented with an epulis that had been removed twice surgically and had returned (**a**). A 5 mm pocket was present on the distal aspect of the UL3, which also tested negative to sensibility testing (**b**). Following root canal treatment and periodontal treatment the periodontal pocket resolved, and the epulis consolidated, but remained (**c**). The patient chose to accept this as surgical removal may have led to recession

Cemental Tears

Clinical signs of cemental tears include deep periodontal pockets, gingival swelling, suppuration, bleeding on probing, bony destruction with periradicular abscesses, recession/attachment loss and tooth mobility. The tooth is often vital and the signs and symptoms do not resolve with endodontic treatment. Fragments may be visible on radiographs and can be misdiagnosed for periodontal lesions, endodontic lesions, root fractures, and perio-endo lesions (Jeng et al. 2018; Ong et al. 2019). It has been reported that fractures of the cementum not exposed to the oral cavity can repair and reattach to the dentine, or drift into the tissues and become fused to the bone (Marquam 2003). It is thought that the outcome of treatment is dictated by the location of the cemental tear and the prognosis of the treatment, with better outcomes if the tear is in the mid or coronal third of the root (Ong et al. 2019).

Case 13 This case demonstrates the difficulties of diagnosing a cemental tear. A 28-year old male presented with external cervical resorption of the LR3 in 2019 (Fig. 7.6a). At this stage the LR3 responded positively to sensibility testing, was not tender to percussion, without associated swelling/sinus/tenderness or deep periodontal pocketing. There was no history of trauma, however, the patient had undergone extensive orthodontic treatment with fixed appliances. The resorption defect was accessible lingually with minimal reflection of the gingival sulcus and was repaired with MTA over the pulp chamber and a glass ionomer cement restoration. The pulp chamber was not encroached by the resorption or the treatment. The tooth continued to test positive to sensibility testing and has ever been tender to percussion. The patient then presented with a swelling in the attached gingivae, distal to the LR3 (Fig. 7.6b, c). It was possible to place a GP point in the sinus and this led to the coronal third of the root on the distal aspect, however, also showed a radiolucent area on the mesial aspect of the LR3 (Fig. 7.6d). Following root

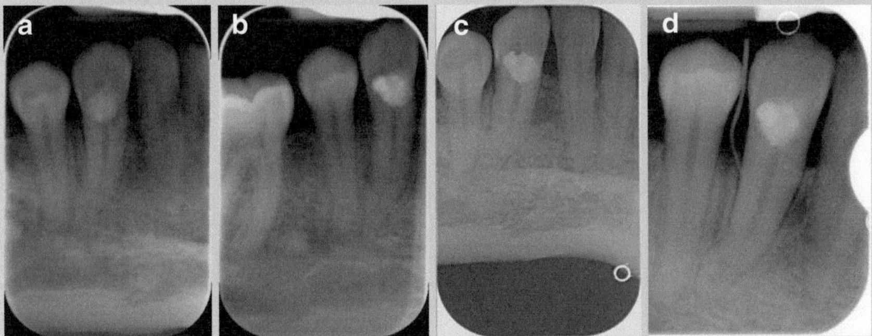

Fig. 7.6 LCPA radiographs of the LR3: (**a**) Review surgical repair of external invasive resorption at the cervical level (August 2019). (**b**) Review in December 2019. (**c**) Review in August 2020. (**d**) Review in October 2020 with a GP point in the buccally draining sinus

surface debridement of the distal aspect of the LR3 and improvement in oral hygiene, the lesion on the distal aspect of the LR3 healed.

CBCT of the LR3 revealed a mesiolingual radiolucency and small fragment of radiopacity (Fig. 7.7), which was assumed to be a possible fragment of retained deciduous root, and the recommendation from the radiology/histopathology meeting was to review and repeat the CBCT at 1 year. The CBCT confirmed the presence of external cervical and apical internal resorption without associated apical pathology. The patient then presented almost a year later with tenderness on the gingival tissues around the LR3, without an associated deep periodontal pocket, the tooth testing positive to sensibility testing and no other clinical signs of infection were seen. A plain film radiograph revealed the enlargement of the radiolucent lesion on the mesial aspect of the LR3 and a more obvious radiopacity (Fig. 7.8a). A diagnosis was difficult to make and it was assumed that there might be some irritation from a fragment of root or endodontic involvement. Surgical debridement of the area was recommended. The patient was keen to avoid surgery but willing to under go root canal treatment of the LR3. When the patient presented for first stage endodontic treatment few months later, he presented with a swelling and sinus within the attached gingivae on the mesio-lingual aspect of the LR3. The

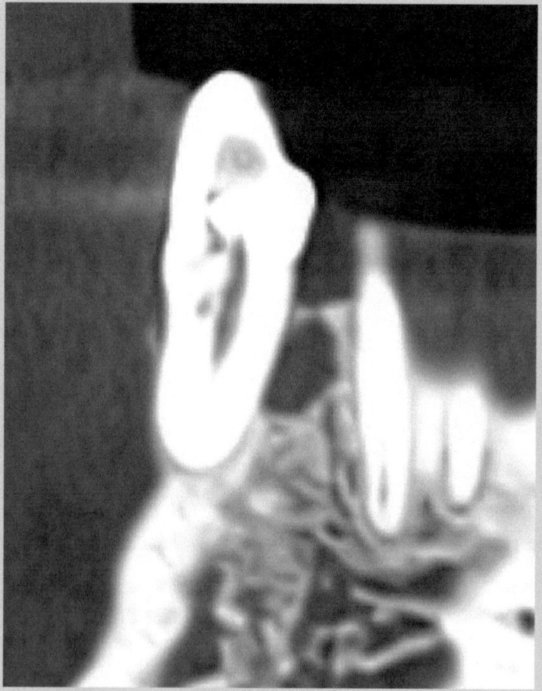

Fig. 7.7 Sagittal image of CBCT (August 2020) showing a radiolucency on the mesial aspect of the root of the LR3

tooth still tested positive to sensibility testing without tenderness to percussion or mobility. A periodontal pocket of 9 mm was present on the mesiolingual line angle of the LR3. A GP point in the sinus led to the mesial aspect of the LR3, where a radiopacity was clearly visible (Fig. 7.8b). Surgical debridement of the area was recommended and the patient warned that endodontic treatment might also be required.

A mucoperiosteal flap was raised buccally and lingually to the LR3, the defect was cleaned and the root surface was debrided with hand and ultrasonic instruments. Little or no calculus was seen. During surgical debridement a three-walled defect was seen on the mesiolingual aspect of the LR3, without extension to the apex of the LR3, and filled with granulation tissue. Microscopic examination did not reveal any fragments of hard tissue and histopathological analysis revealed granulation tissue and not the presence of any hard dental tissues. The patient is currently asymptomatic and under review. It would be of advantage to avoid endodontic treatment unless necessary, as there are added complications of finding the canal coronally as it may have retreated since repair of the resorption defect, the curvature of the root

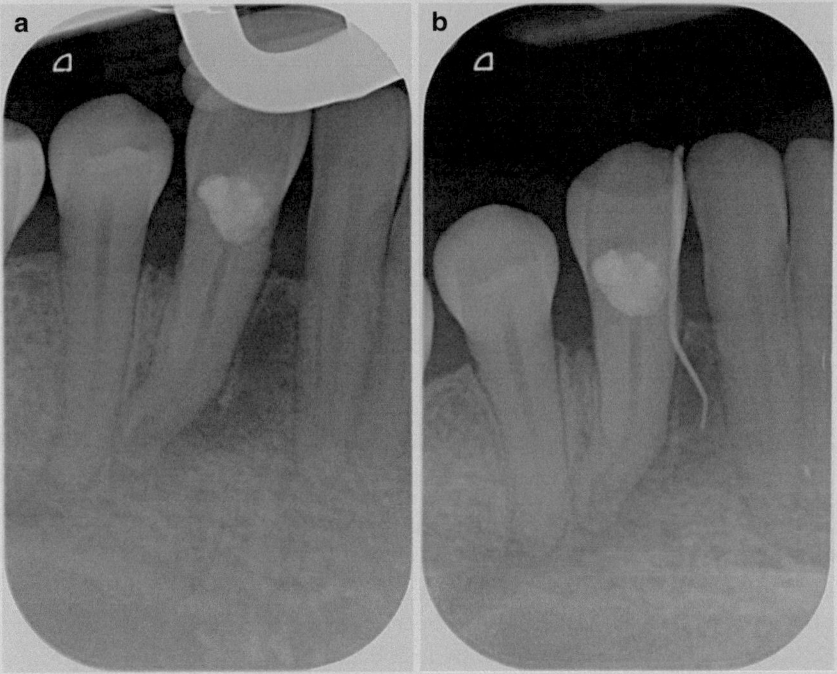

Fig. 7.8 LCPA radiographs of LR3: (**a**) Progression of the mesial radiolucency associated with the mesial aspect of the root of the LR3 (July 2021). (**b**) With a GP point in the lingual sinus tracking to the mesial radiolucency associated with the LR3 (September 2021)

and the presence of apical internal resorption. The periodontal pocket has resolved, the LR3 remains not tender to percussion, with normal responses to sensibility testing. The associated radiolucency has been reducing with maintenance of the bone coronal to the lesion (Fig. 7.9a, b). Good oral hygiene has helped to prevent re-establishment of the periodontal pocket. One could argue that the LR3 should undergo non-surgical endodontic treatment in any event, to arrest the internal resorptive process in the apical third of the canal, however, the patients opted not to pursue this in case of flare up of an otherwise asymptomatic tooth.

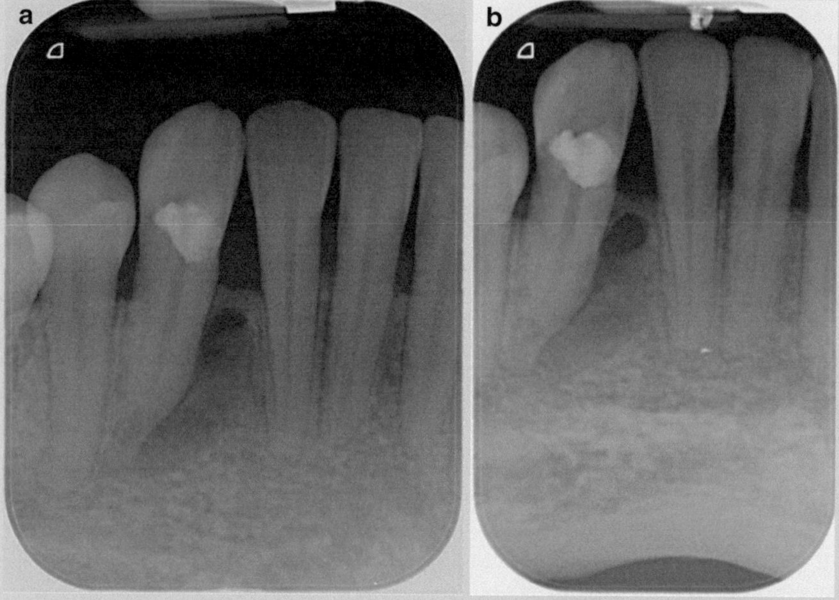

Fig. 7.9 LCPA radiographs of LR3: (**a**) Reduction of the mesial radiolucency associated with the mesial aspect of the root of the LR3 in July 2022). (**b**) at review in July 2023

A Case to Illustrate the Management of Periodontal Disease with Endodontic Manifestations

Treatment of periodontal disease has been described previously. If the primary cause is periodontal, with a periodontal lesion that is progressing, then periodontal treatment (root surface debridement and oral hygiene instructions) is indicated. The diagnosis may only be ascertained correctly once the treatment for periodontal disease has been completed: a lesion of periodontal origin will resolve with periodontal treatment alone. Case 14 demonstrates a primarily periodontal lesion, and difficulty establishing endodontic involvement. This is especially the case in multi-rooted teeth, where sensibility testing may not reveal the true vitality of each canal.

Case 14 A 36-year-old male patient presented with localised periodontal disease associated with the UL2 and LR6 (Fig. 7.10). The patient was excellent with his oral hygiene, using snug fitting interdental brushes horizontally in all areas and also gently using interdental brushes vertically in the mesial pockets of the LR6, as well as using a modified single tufted brush. As healing occurs, the interdental brushes used horizontally may need to be replaced with larger diameter brushes, however, vertical interdental brushes should be replaced with thinner diameter brushes, and ideally extending to a shallower pocket. Patients should be informed of this change to avoid damage to periodontal pockets. The UL2 showed healing with non-surgical periodontal treatment, and although the LR6 showed some improvement, a deep pocket remained. In December 2018, it was difficult to make a decision as to whether the LR6 required root canal treatment (Fig. 7.11a, b). A decision was made not to carry out root canal treatment after taking a periapical radiograph with a gutta percha point in the pocket (Fig. 7.11c), as it did not track to the apex of the mesial roots. Open flap debridement was performed with regeneration using a synthetic scaffolding material without the need for a membrane (Fig. 7.11d). During surgery it was possible to see that the apex of the mesial roots were not involved in the periodontal lesion. Following regenerative periodontal surgery, the mesial pocket reduced and bony infill was seen (Fig. 7.11e, f).

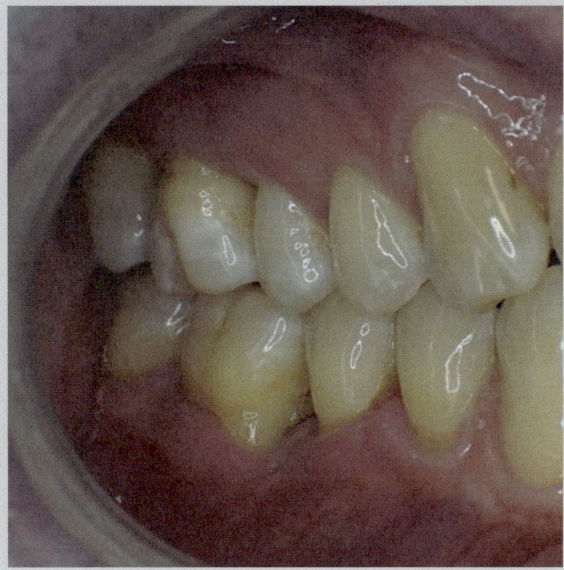

Fig. 7.10 Intra-oral photograph of the LR6 demonstrating excellent oral hygiene and recession along the mesial aspect of the LR6

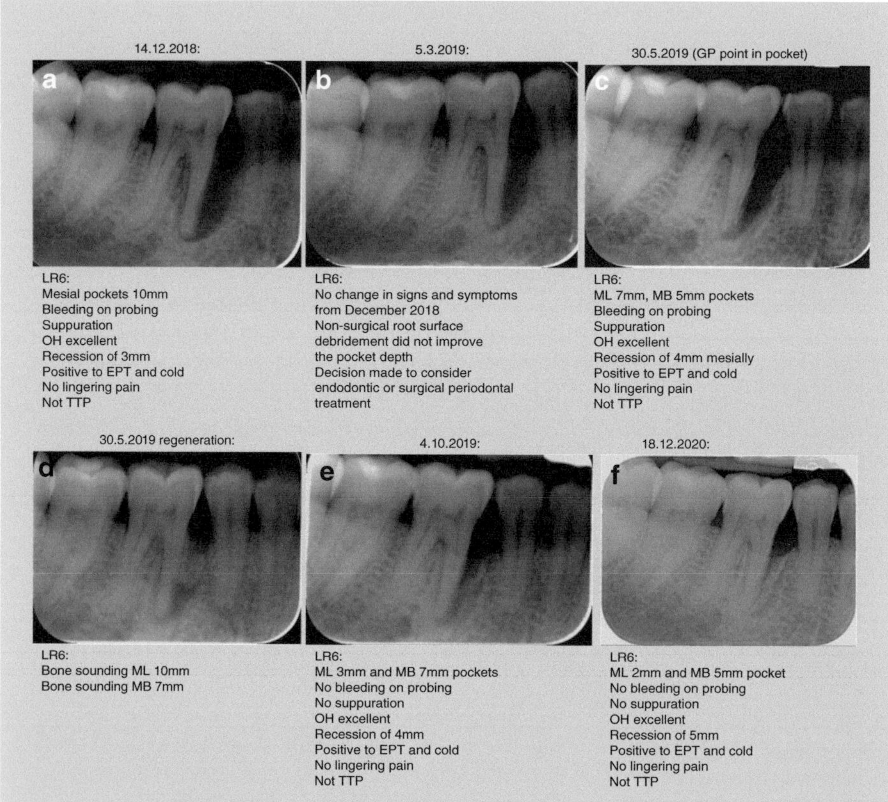

Fig. 7.11 LCPA radiographs of LR6 at various time points. (**a**) Remaining mesial deep pocket and radiolucency following non-surgical periodontal treatment. (**b**) No improvement with further non-surgical periodontal treatment. (**c**) GP point in the deep pocket tracked to the base of periodontal pocket. (**d**) Post-regenerative periodontal surgery. (**e** and **f**) Follow-up radiographs

Future plan: supportive periodontal care with 3 monthly, full periodontal indices, sensibility testing, debridement of pockets that are 4 mm of deeper under local anaesthetic (2 minutes per site) and oral hygiene instructions.

Learning point: Placing a gutta percha point into a solitary pocket before taking a long cone periapical radiograph may help to determine whether the apex of a root is involved in the lesion.

Diagnosis of these periodontal lesions with manifestations of endodontic disease can be difficult. When in doubt, periodontal disease should be managed with improvement in oral hygiene, removal of the exacerbating factors such as overhangs and root surface debridement, followed by periodontal re-assessment. There may be a need for further non-surgical or surgical periodontal treatment. Those teeth with possible endodontic involvement should undergo sensibility testing and radiographic review as part of the periodontal re-assessment. If and when there are signs of loss of vitality, endodontic treatment should be sought. Performing periodontal treatment only in a true combined lesion may lead to initial healing of the periodontal pocket, however, the periodontal pocket will return if the source of infection from the pulp is not managed. Therefore, when a periodontal pocket fails to heal, pulpal necrosis should be investigated, prior to considering surgical periodontal treatment.

References

Abbott PV, Salgado JC. Strategies for the endodontic management of concurrent endodontic and periodontal diseases. Aust Dent J. 2009;54:S70–85.

Al-Hezaimi K, Naghshbandi J, Simon JH, Rotstein I. Successful treatment of a radicular groove by intentional replantation and Emdogain therapy: four years follow- up. Oral Surg Oral Med Oral Pathol Oral Radiol Endod. 2009;107:82–5.

Bergenholtz G, Lindhe J. Effect of experimentally induced marginal periodontitis and periodontal scaling on the dental pulp. J Clin Periodontol. 1978;5:59–73.

Chapple ILC, Lumley PJ. The perio-endo interface. Dent Update. 1999;26:331–41.

Fonseca GM, Fonseca RM, Cantín M. Massive fibrous epulis-a case report of a 10-year-old lesion. Int J Oral Sci. 2014;6(3):182–4.

Herrera D, Retamal-Valdes B, Alonso B, Feres M. Acute periodontal lesions (periodontal abscesses and necrotizing periodontal diseases) and endo-periodontal lesions. J Periodontol. 2018;89(Suppl 1):S85–S102.

Jeng P-Y, Pitarch ALLRM, Chang M-C, Wu Y-H, Jeng J-H. Cemental tear: to know what we have neglected in dental practice. J Formos Med Assoc. 2018;117(4):261–7.

Kogon SL. The prevalence, location and conformation of palato-radicular grooves in maxillary incisors. J Periodontol. 1986;57:231–4.

Langeland K. Tissue response to dental caries. Endodont Dent Traumatol. 1987;3:149–71.

Langeland K, Rodrigues H, Dowden W. Periodontal disease, bacteria, and pulpal histopathology. Oral Surg Oral Med Oral Pathol. 1974;37:257–70.

Lara VS, Consolaro A, Bruce RS. Macroscopic and microscopic analysis of the palato-gingival groove. J Endod. 2000;26:345–50.

Lindhe J, Lang NP, Karring T. Clinical periodontology and implant dentistry. Oxford: Blackwell Munksgaard; 2008.

Marquam BJ. Atypical localised deep pocket die to a cemental tear: case report. J Contemp Dent Pract. 2003;4(3):52–64.

Ong TK, Harun N, Lim TW. Cemental tear on maxillary anterior incisors: a description of clinical, radiographic, and histopathological features of two clinical cases. Eur Endod J. 2019;4:90–5.

Seltzer S, Bender IB. Inflammation in the odontoblastic layer of the dental pulp. J Am Dent Assoc. 1959;59:720–4.

Withers JA, Brunsvold MA, Killoy WJ, Rahe AJ. The relationship of palato-gingival grooves to localized periodontal disease. J Periodontol. 1981;52:41–4.

Zehnder M, Gold SI, Hasselgren G. Pathologic interaction in pulpal and periodontal tissues. J Clin Periodontol. 2002;29:663–71.

Endodontic Infections That May Have Periodontal Manifestations

8

Abstract

This chapter discusses lesions of endodontic origin, which develop periodontal manifestations and present as 'endo-perio' lesions.

Endodontics Lesions with Periodontal Manifestations

Pulpitis never or very rarely causes a periodontal lesion. In the presence of inflammation as a result of loss of pulp vitality, if the cementum is intact, any microbial products within the dentinal tubules are unable to reach the periodontal ligament. Once the pulp starts to become infected, there is further inflammation, which may reach the periapical or periradicular tissues. This inflammation could be silent and asymptomatic, maybe stable over many years and may only be diagnosed radiographically (Abbott 2004). These lesions therefore, may appear apically or as periradicular lesions, where there are large lateral canals or furcation canals. Long standing infections can lead to drainage through the periodontal architecture, and lead to localised periodontal disease. Case 15 describes a case where a lateral peri-radicular lesion failed to heal after non-surgical endodontic treatment and the cause may only be known after surgical exploration.

S. Eliyas, *The Periodontic-Endodontic Interface*, https://doi.org/10.1007/978-3-031-49937-1_8

Case 15 A 63-year-old male patient presented with a non-vital LR2, with tenderness to biting as well as percussion, and an intermittent sinus draining from the buccal aspect of the attached gingivae adjacent to the LR2 (Fig. 8.1). No deep periodontal pockets were present. During root canal treatment a second or large lateral canal was not found (Fig. 8.2a). The tooth was asymptomatic for 18 months after which the signs and symptoms of periradicular periodontitis returned (Fig. 8.2b). CBCT examination of the LR2 confirmed the presence of distal periradicular radiolucency, however, failed to show the presence of a second or large lateral canal. Careful examination of the CBCT did reveal a possible groove in the root in the area of the periradicular radiolucency (Fig. 8.3). This demonstrates the difficulties with diagnosis of such lesions. It is likely that there is a biofilm of bacteria on the root surface and access is only possible surgically.

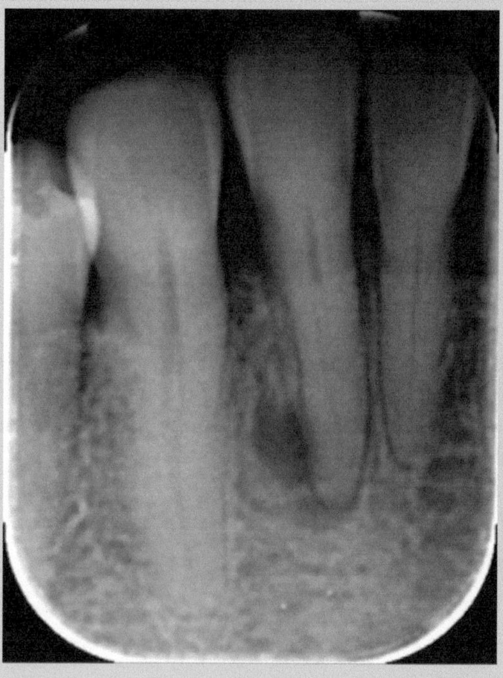

Fig. 8.1 LCPA pre-operative radiograph of the LR2 showing 20% bone loss and a peri-radicular radiolucency associated with the apical third of the root of the LR2

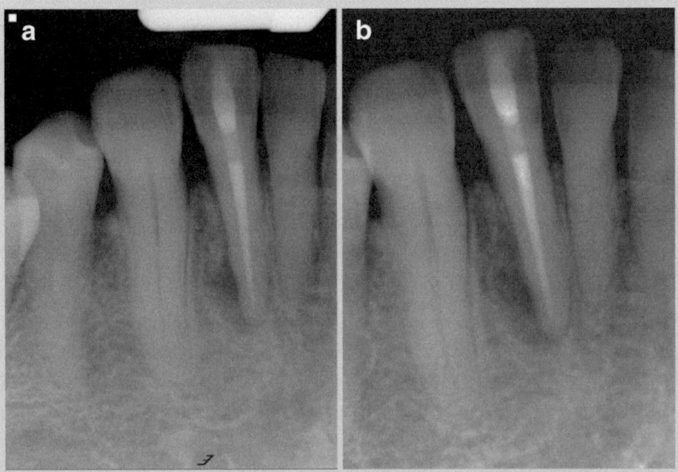

Fig. 8.2 LCPA radiograph of the LR2 (**a**) immediately post root canal treatment and (**b**) at annual review

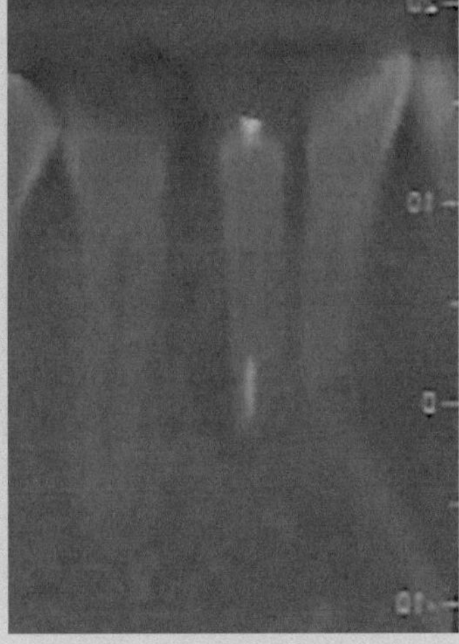

Fig. 8.3 CBCT of the LR2 confirmed the presence of a radiolucency in the apical third of the roots, however a fracture line or second canal were not found (the quality of the CBCT is not ideal)

Inflammation of the pulp could also be acute with throbbing pain, tenderness to percussion and palpation, be associated with increased tooth mobility as well as apical and marginal swelling. Such symptoms can also occur with aggressive periodontitis, root perforations, root fractures and root resorption. When pulpal disease causes inflammation beyond the tooth, there is an effect on the periodontal tissues but can also result in bone, cementum and dentine resorption (Hargreaves et al. 2011).

Periapical or periradicular disease has previously been classified (World Health Organisation 1995; Nair 1997). Teeth with endodontic infections may manifest as acute or chronic apical abscesses. Pressure of exudate within the tissues will result in tissue destruction as a path of drainage is sought. Acute apical abscesses may present as a swelling intra orally or extra orally, with or without a draining sinus. A chronic apical abscess is a localised collection of pus with a draining sinus. Chronic apical abscesses may drain though a sinus intraorally or extraorally depending on the position of the apical foramina in relation to muscle attachments (Fig. 5.2). Infections spreading along facial planes can lead to life-threatening facial cellulitis, Ludwig's Angina, orbital cellulitis, cavernous sinus thrombosis, mediastinitis, actinomycosis, osteomyelitis and septicaemia (Abbott 2004). Clinically, these could manifest as extreme pain, severe swelling, fever, malaise, lymphadenopathy, mobility of the tooth and tenderness to percussion or even light touching of the tooth. Radiographically, a peri-radicular lesion may or may not be evident. Table 8.1 summarises a useful and practical classification of periradicular disease of endodontic origin (Abbott 2004).

Usually, the presence of an apical area seen radiographically is a result of bacteria within the canal (intra-radicular infection), however, can be persistent if there is extra-radicular colonization of microbes (Nair 2006). Apical areas could also be as a result of foreign body reactions, the presence of cholesterol crystals, the presence of true cysts, or as a result of scar tissue formation during healing (Nair 2006). Chronic apical abscesses are usually not uncomfortable, unless an acute exacerbation occurs, which is when the sinus tract heals while pus continues to be produced and then traps within the deep tissues (Abbott and Salgado 2009). Intra oral draining of a sinus maybe seen within the sulcus reflection, within the attached gingivae, sometimes draining near the gingival crevice or draining through a periodontal pocket (Fig. 8.4). Intrapulpal infection can promote epithelial downgrowth along denuded dentine surfaces (Blomlöf et al. 1988; Blomlöf 1993; Jansson and Ehnevid 1998). Single rooted teeth with apical radiolucencies have been associated with deeper periodontal pockets, more attachment loss as seen radiographically, and less of a reduction of periodontal pockets after treatment, when compared to teeth without endodontic infections (Zehnder et al. 2002).

Table 8.1 Periapical disease may present in various forms (Abbott 2004)

Periapical disease	Description	Clinical Signs	Radiographic signs
Acute periradicular periodontitis	An acute inflammation of the periodontal ligament space, and can be as a result of occlusal trauma, trauma from endodontic instruments or as a result of pulpal disease and non-vitality. Bacterial infection or toxins may have invaded the periodontal ligament space	Spontaneous pain Hypersensitive to heat and relived by application of cold Tenderness to percussion May or may not response to EPT/cold testing	Widened periodontal ligament space without the presence of an apical area
Chronic periradicular periodontitis	Infection of the periodontal ligament space. Acute exacerbation of chronic apical periodontitis may present as pain and swelling (Phoenix abscess)	Usually no clinical symptoms Not usually tender to bite on, however may 'feel different' upon percussion testing No response to EPT/cold/heat	Apical radiolucency seen radiographically Occasionally occur as a condensing osteitis
Periradicular abscess (acute)	Purulent breakdown and the presence of pus within the apical tissues	Very painful to biting pressure, percussion and palpation No response to sensibility testing Varying degrees of mobility Swelling and buccal tenderness +/− febrile and cervical lymphadenopathy	Apical radiolucency seen radiographically
Periradicular abscess (chronic) or suppurative periradicular periodontitis	Purulent breakdown and the presence of pus intermittently draining via a sinus tract	Asymptomatic No response to sensibility testing Not particularly tender to percussion, however may 'feel different'	Apical radiolucency seen radiographically

Peri-radicular cysts—often considered forms of chronic apical periodontitis, and may have the same manifestations as above. Most lesions seen radiographically are not cysts and 85% of these heal with endodontic treatment. Of the remaining 15%, 6% are pocket cysts and 9% are true cysts (Nair et al. 1996). A periapical pocket cyst is an epithelium-lined lesion that communicates with the root canal system, and therefore, provision of root canal treatment is likely to lead to healing. A periapical true cyst is an epithelium lined lesion without communication with the root canal system, and therefore, will not heal with endodontic treatment. Cysts can only be diagnosed from histological examinations

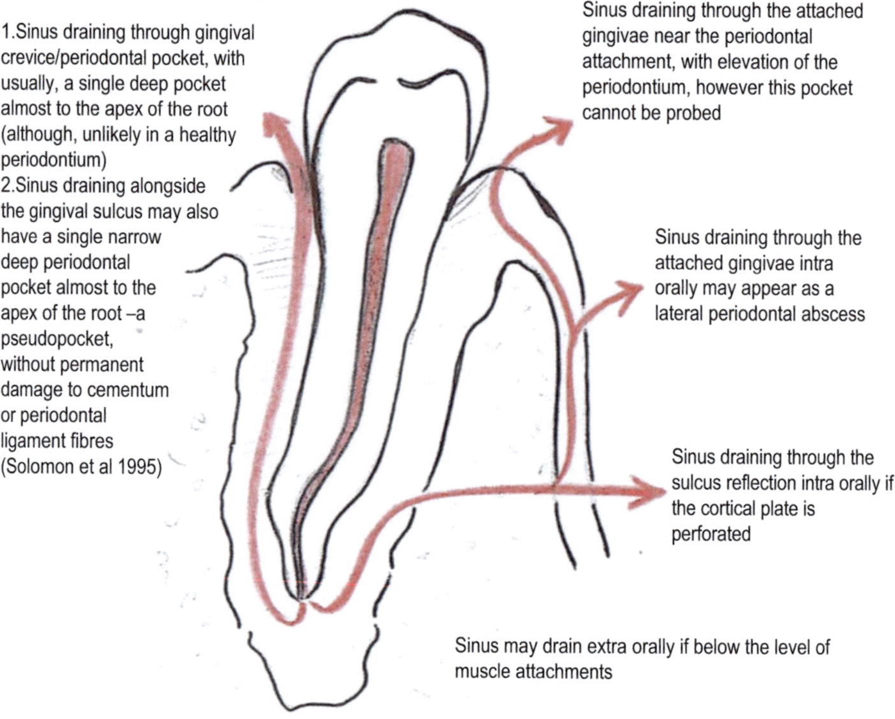

Fig. 8.4 The intraoral draining of periradicular periodontitis

When endodontic infections drain through a periodontal pocket, careful probing is required to find the pocket, and often it may be possible to probe almost to apex of the root with no other pockets being present around the tooth. This may be difficult to distinguish from a periodontal pocket or pocket associated with a fracture within the root or perforation as it often presents as a deep, narrow periodontal pocket (Fig. 8.5). Draining through a healthy periodontal ligament is however unusual (Abbott and Salgado 2009). Multi-rooted teeth can drain into the furcation area presenting like a 'through and through' furcation involvement. Furcation bone loss may also be seen if endodontic infections are communicating via accessory canals, perforations or fractures in the floor of the pulp chamber. These accessory canals adjacent to such furcation radiolucencies or adjacent to periradicular radiolucencies may only be visible after completion of root filling when sealer may enter the accessory canals. If these radiolucencies are of endodontic origin, these bony lesions will fill in after successful endodontic treatment.

Pulpal degeneration results in necrotic debris and bacterial byproducts/toxic irritants that can move down the canal, towards the apex, through the apical foramen and potentially cause periodontal destruction apically, and possibly migrate

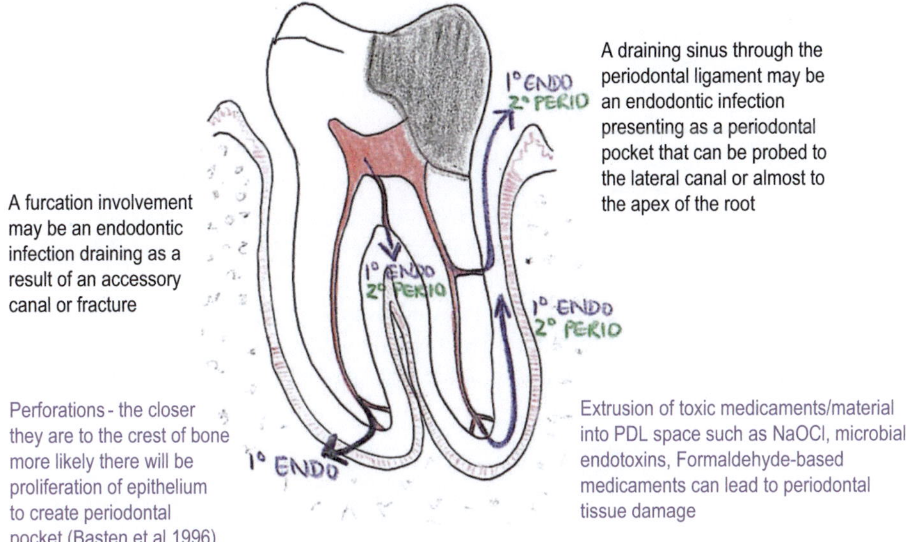

Fig. 8.5 Primary endodontic lesions leading to periodontal involvement and therefore, secondary periodontal manifestations

towards the gingival margin. However, endo-perio lesions are rare, considering that there are a lot of teeth with apical periodontitis which do not develop into periodontal pockets. The presence of necrotic debris and irritants could stimulate osteoclastic activity and may encourage or aggravate periodontal pocket formation and bone loss, as well as impair wound healing to accelerate periodontal disease progression. This is also possible with endodontic medicaments. The extent of the destruction depends on the virulence of the microbes, toxicity of the medication, duration of the disease, the presence of a foreign body reaction and the host's defense mechanisms.

Primary endodontic lesions resorb bone apically and laterally, destroying the attachment adjacent to the non-vital tooth. This may lead to pain, tenderness of the tooth to pressure or percussion, increased tooth mobility, swelling of the marginal gingivae or the presence of a sinus (either through the bone or through the periodontal ligament space with a narrow isolated deep pocket with or without suppuration). It is always worthwhile placing a GP point in the sinus and taking a long cone periapical radiograph. In the furcation area, bone loss may appear as a furcation III defect (Ramfjord and Ash 1979). Electric pulp testing may reveal an abnormal response or no response indicating a necrotic pulp. Treatment required is endodontic only, and the pocket should be healed at the 3-month review. Sometimes the results of sensibility testing can be confusing even in single rooted teeth (Case 16).

Case 16 In this case, the patient presented with a buccal swelling in the attached gingivae of the UL1, with an associated pocket of 3 mm. The tooth was not tender to percussion, there was no tenderness or swelling over the apex of the UL1, and gave a positive response to sensibility testing. The UL1 was diagnosed as a lateral periodontal abscess, as there was a developmental groove buccally, in an otherwise periodontally sound patient (Fig. 8.6a). The UL1 was initially treated with non-surgical periodontal treatment, which did not resolve the buccal swelling. The tooth tested negative to sensibility testing 5 months later, and developed an apical area, as seen radiographically. Endodontic treatment was performed and the tooth was non-vital on entry (Fig. 8.6b). The buccal swelling and pocket resolved, the apical radiolucency seen radiographically resolved and the tooth remains asymptomatic (Fig. 8.6c).

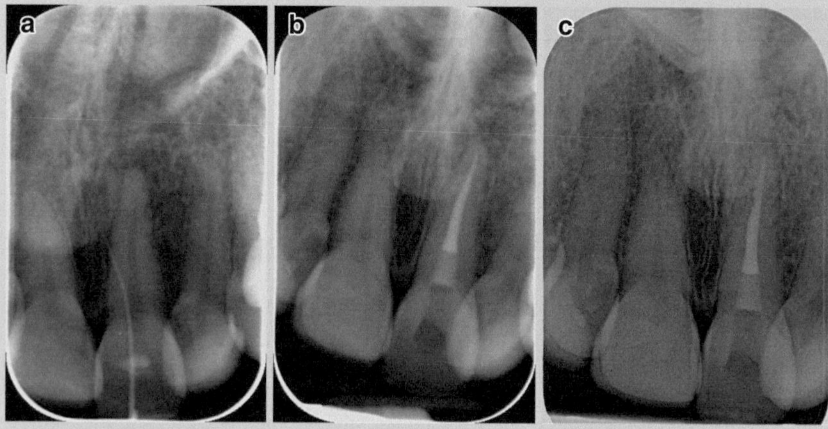

Fig. 8.6 LCPA radiograph of the UL1 (**a**) with a GP point in the periodontal pocket (March 2019), (**b**). following completion of root canal treatment (March 2020) and (**c**) at follow-up (March 2021)

Primary endodontic lesions that are untreated may cause an accumulation of plaque and calculus in the sinus tract, leading to apical migration of epithelium and attachment, resulting in a persistent periodontal pocket. In addition to sensibility tests suggesting a necrotic pulp, there will also be a long standing periodontal pocket with plaque and calculus present, with a possible radiographic appearance of a vertical or angular bone defect adjacent to the non-vital tooth. In such a case, both endodontic and periodontal treatment (root surface debridement of the periodontal pocket) would be required (Cases 17 and 18).

Case 17 The UL4 presented with a swelling in the buccal attached gingivae, with a healing sinus. It was not possible to place a gutta percha point in the sinus as the patient had recently taken antibiotics and the sinus had drained. A mid-buccal pocket of 9 mm was present; the UL4 was grade II mobile and exhibited fremitus (Fig. 8.7a). The UL4 and UL5 were tender to percussion. The UL5 had been restored with a crown and might appear the most likely to lose vitality, however, the UL4 tested negative to sensibility testing. The results from the use of a Tooth Slooth were inconclusive as both the UL4 and UL5 were tender to bite on, with no altered sensation on release. Radiographic examination revealed a diffuse apical area around the root of the UL4 (Fig. 8.7b). It was difficult to explain why this tooth with a small disto-occlusal restoration lost vitality.

The decision was taken to commence root canal treatment on the UL4. Both canals were non-vital on entry and first stage of root canal treatment was completed with root surface debridement of the mid-buccal pocket. The patient was advised to use a small interdental brush gently, vertically in the pocket. The patient was informed that as the pocket will heal by a reduction in depth and width, which will determine how far the brush could be inserted. Soon after eliminating the necrotic/infected pulp and cleaning of the pocket, the swelling, sinus, mobility, fremitus and tenderness to bite on resolved (Fig. 8.8a, b). Between appointments, the patient presented 2 weeks after first stage of endodontics with the palatal cusp of the UL4 having fractured horizontally at gingival level (Fig. 8.9a). This is likely to have been the cause of the UL4 losing vitality, as the disto-occlusal restoration was not close to the pulp chamber. The tooth was deemed restorable with a post core and three quarter crown (Fig. 8.9b, c).

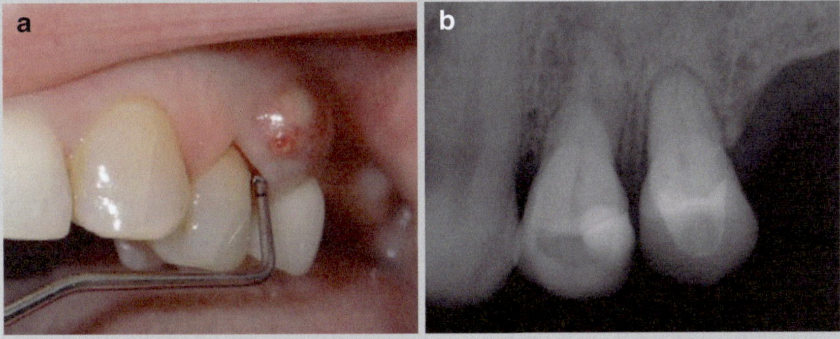

Fig. 8.7 (a) Photograph of the UL4 showing a swelling in the attached gingivae with an associated single deep periodontal pocket and (b) LCPA pre-operative radiograph of the UL4

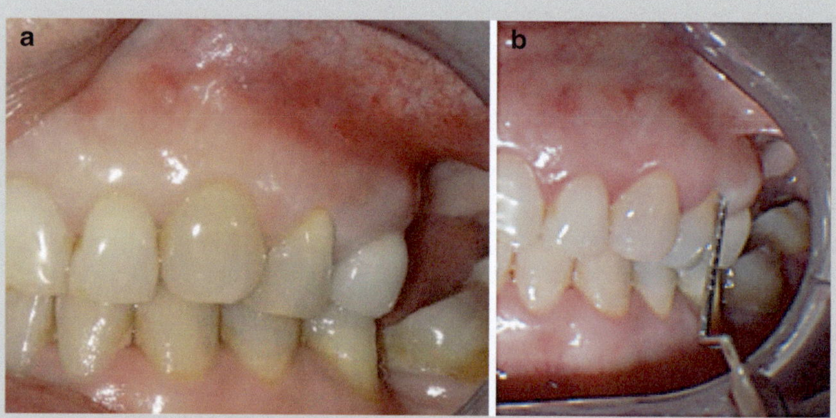

Fig. 8.8 (**a**) Photograph of the UL2 after the first stage of root canal treatment (buccal swelling and sinus resolved). (**b**) Photograph of the UL4 showing resolution of the periodontal pocket

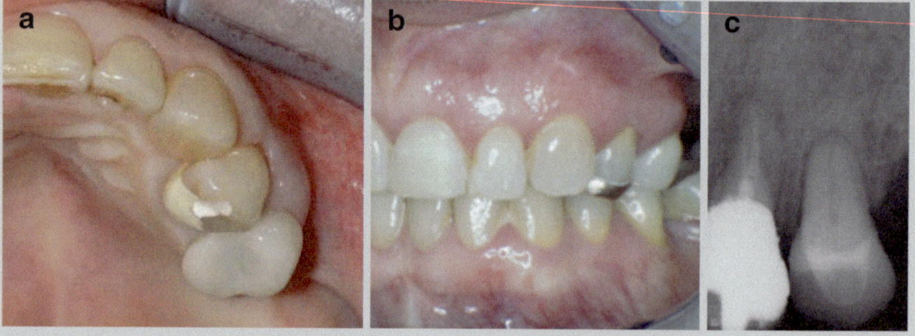

Fig. 8.9 (**a**) Photograph of the UL4 following repair of the fractured palatal cusp. (**b**) Photograph of the UL4 following restoration. (**c**) LCPA radiograph of the UL4

A causal relationship between endodontic infections and periodontal disease is not yet established, as periodontal pockets of endodontic origin will resolve with endodontic treatment. However, pulpal disease can initiate or maintain periodontal disease (Czarnecki and Schilder 1979). When healthy pulps were compared to endodontically treated teeth, teeth that were endodontically treated showed increased pocket probing depths, more marginal breakdown and retarded/impaired periodontal tissue healing subsequent to periodontal therapy (Jansson et al. 1993; Ehnevid et al. 1993). Therefore, endodontic retreatment should be adjunct to periodontal treatment in these cases. Although some research has shown that the periodontal tissues may regenerate better in those teeth that have not required root canal treatment (Sanders et al. 1983), other studies have shown that the ability to regenerate is unaffected by the status of the pulp (Perlmutter et al. 1987; Diem et al. 1974), with the ability of the cementum to be laid down being unaffected by extruded filling material, especially if the material is MTA (Naik et al. 2014). There has been a suggestion that endodontic treatment is completed before root surface debridement to ensure that periodontal reattachment does occur (Harrington 1979; Blomlöf et al. 1988).

Case 18 A 64-year-old female presented with a buccally draining sinus in the attached gingivae, close to the gingival margin of the LR6, without an associated deep periodontal pocket (depth of 2 mm). A true endodontic lesion draining through the attached gingivae close to the gingival crevice. When a gutta percha point was placed in the sinus, it tracked to the distal root (Fig. 8.10a–c). The first periapical radiograph revealed a furcation involvement and possible furcal perforation in one of the mesial roots, which may be the cause of the buccally draining sinus. However, careful examination of the radiograph does show a distal peri-radicular radiolucency associated with the distal root. The second radiograph at a different angle revealed this not to be the case (Fig. 8.11a, b). This case highlights the importance of placing a gutter percha point whenever possible, and the importance of taking more than one radiograph, at a different angle. Although the full length of the silver points could not be removed, the finding, negotiating and cleaning of a missed distal canal resolved the sinus within weeks of starting treatment (Fig. 8.12a, b). Complete healing was present clinically and visible radiographically at 1-year follow-up (Fig. 8.12c).

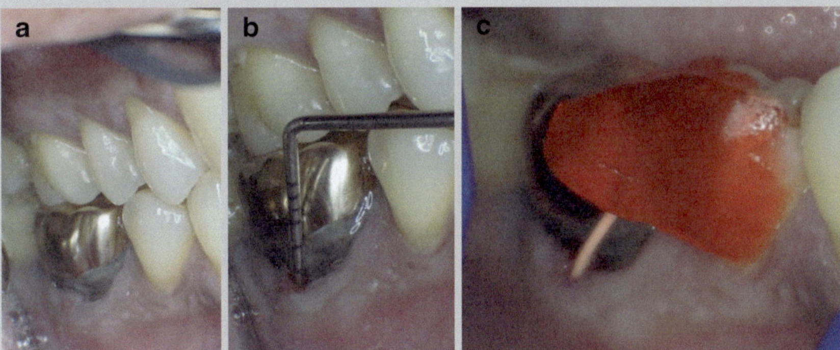

Fig. 8.10 (**a**) Pre-operative photograph of the LR6 restored with a gold crown. (**b**) Photograph of the LR6 showing the absence of a deep periodontal pocket. (**c**) GP point in the draining buccal sinus adjacent to the gingival margin, secured in place with ribbon wax

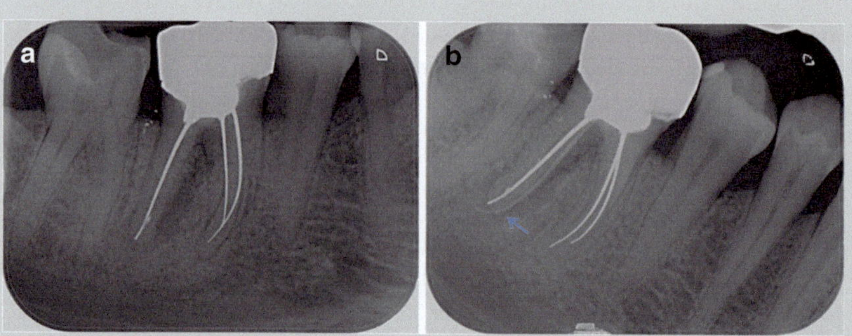

Fig. 8.11 (**a**) LCPA radiograph of the LR6 showing the presence of a peri-radicular radiolucency associated with the distal root of the LR6. (**b**) LCPA radiograph of the LR6 with a GP point in the sinus tracking to the distal root

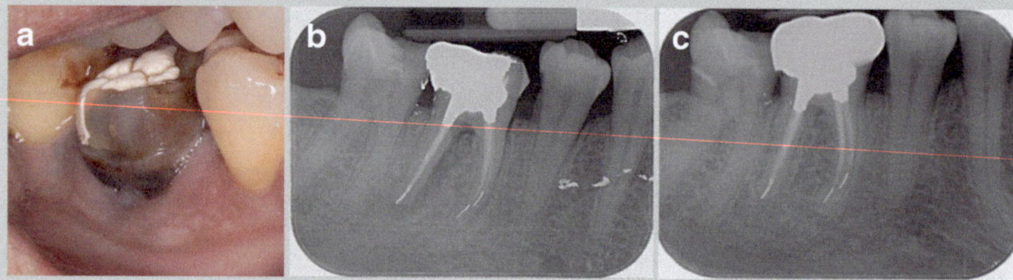

Fig. 8.12 (**a**) Photograph of the LR6 showing resolution of the buccally draining sinus after commencement of root canal treatment. (**b**). LCPA radiograph of the LR6 following completion of root canal treatment (it was not possible to remove the apical portions of the silver points). (**c**) LCPA radiograph of the LR6 showing healing at annual review

Endodontic treatment itself can also cause periodontal tissue damage. Acute toxic and allergic reactions to high concentrations of sodium hypochlorite, and previous use of arsenic or formaldehyde-based medications used to devitalise pulps can cause periodontal breakdown. Medicaments used in the canal can irritate periodontal tissues, and the level of irritation will depend on the medication, presence of microbes and the host defence system. Extrusion of toxic medicaments or root canal fillings into the periodontium during endodontic treatment may cause an inflammatory reaction (Ricucci and Langeland 1998), however, often these extrusion of obturation materials do not cause long lasting pain or periodontal breakdown unless there is microbial infection as well (Chapple and Lumley 1999).

Root canal perforations, strip perforations and post related perforations are possible and compromise periodontal health. Root fracture or crack development could also lead to periodontal tissue damage. More coronally placed fractures and perforations (in the coronal third of the root) may cause a localised deep pocket, however, those in the apical or mid third of the root may not. Iatrogenic lesions as a result of root perforations, fractures and extruded obturation materials, may result in resorption of the cementum and communication with between the pulpal and periodontal tissues. Iatrogenic lesions can be more complex to treat.

Perforations

The outcome may be compromised where there are perforations (Farzaneh et al. 2004; Ng et al. 2011; Fuss and Trope 1996). Perforations are often diagnosed with profuse bleeding within the canal during treatment (as with some resorptive defects) and when aberrant apex locator readings occur. Strip perforations are difficult to diagnose and repair. 'Minimally invasive endodontics' may result in a reduction in perforations. The outcome of perforation repairs depend on the size of the perforation, the position of the perforation in relation to the gingival sulcus, speed of identification and treatment of the perforation, ability to achieve a satisfactory seal, microbial colonisation, accessibility to treatment of the remaining canal and the chance of building a new attachment as well as presence of a concomitant periodontal pocket (Clauder and Shin 2009; Fuss and Trope 1996).

A 'critical zone' for perforations has been identified as level of the crestal bone and epithelial attachment. Perforations coronal to this zone will have a good prognosis as access to repair is good, and perforations can be orthodontically moved out of this zone to improve prognosis (Fuss and Trope 1996). Perforations at the level of the alveolar crest have a poorer prognosis due to the difficulty of sealing the lesion without microbial ingress and washing away of the sealing material. The closer the perforation is to the crest of bone, the more likelihood of proliferation of the epithelium at the perforation site leading to a deep pocket with or without suppuration, which is more difficult to eliminate (Blomlöf et al. 1988; Christie and Holthuis 1990). Perforations in the coronal third have been shown to be least likely to heal because cell rests of Mallasez proliferate along the periodontal ligament and prevent further bone deposition and regeneration of the periodontal apparatus (Strömberg et al. 1972). Sulcular epithelium migrates below the level of the epithelium. Sometimes there is growth of granulation tissue into the perforation, as the fibroblasts of the periodontal ligament cannot differentiate into odontoblasts like the fibroblasts of the pulp can. Furcal perforations are considered coronal perforations due to their proximity to the epithelial attachment.

Perforations in the middle or apical third of the root (i.e. apical to the critical zone) have the best chance of healing and may be accessible through the canal system, with a better prognosis if adequate sealing is possible (Nicholls 1962). If the perforation is apical to the alveolar crest, there may be sinus with or without periodontal pocket formation (as it may take a longer time for the pocket to form). Perforations can have a good prognosis if they can be sealed from within the canal, however, access to perforations this way can be very difficult. The presence of periodontal involvement lowers the prognosis for a successful repair and healing (Clauder and Shin 2009). In the absence of a periodontal pocket, non-surgical endodontic treatment is indicated, although, surgical repair may also be required.

Treatment of perforations will depend on the position of the perforation. Careful irrigation is recommended where a perforation is suspected, as irrigation is required to reduce the bacterial load. Apically positioned perforations may automatically be filled during the obturation process. Obturation of the canal and perforation as soon as possible is preferable to prevent granulation tissue formation and wound infection (Fuss and Trope 1996). Perforations that are more coronal may require separate sealing before completion of the root canal treatment. Non-healing may warrant surgical repair of the perforation. When perforations are managed quickly, they will not lead to established periodontal inflammation and damage. Long-standing perforations and infections mean poorer potential for repair. Non-surgical perforation repair may be preferable as surgical repair often results in persistent pocket formation and furcation involvement, and in the aesthetic zone, it may lead to recession. In multi-rooted teeth it may be wise to consider hemi-section or root amputation if there is a perforated root rather than extraction of the tooth.

Many materials are available for the repair of perforations. Amalgam, zinc oxide based materials and gutta percha lead to inflammation, with eugenol irritating the tissues. Calcium hydroxide based materials may help to form a bridge of dentine. Glass ionomer cements are biocompatible. Composite restorations require excellent moisture control, which can be difficult in areas with perforations. Materials such as MTA may provide additional cell repair advantages that may promote healing (Ford et al. 1995). MTA is able to promote regeneration of cementum and periodontal apparatus, and requires the presence of moisture to set, however, this takes several hours. Fresh MTA is thought to initially cause cell death, but this is not the case when set. Once set, MTA is osteoconductive (Torabinerjad et al. 1993; Ford et al. 1995; Clauder and Shin 2009). MTA can be white or grey, and grey MTA can discolour teeth. Other biocompatible calcium sulfate materials are available (Parirokh et al. 2018; Torabinerjad et al. 2018). In delayed treatment of perforations extrusion of material is possible. In immediate perforation repair, the periodontal ligament prevents extrusion. Teeth with extruded materials may require surgical intervention to remove the foreign particles from the tissues. In the presence of a concomitant periodontal pocket, once the perforation has been sealed, non-surgical or surgical periodontal treatment will also be required. If the perforation is into an existing periodontal pocket, periodontal treatment will be required after repair of the perforation (Chapple and Lumley 1999).

During surgical repair of perforations and resorption defects, root surface conditioning using 50% citric acid (2–3 minutes) or 15–24% EDTA (2 minutes) or tetracycline (30 s) may be appropriate for materials other than MTA. Guided tissue regeneration may be an option where there is a chance that epithelium downgrowth will prevent periodontal ligament and osseous regeneration. Healing around perforations is likely to be repair rather than regeneration, and therefore, may always appear as a widened periodontal ligament on radiographs (Chapple and Lumley 1999).

All perforations may render teeth with a more guarded prognosis, however, the outcome will depend on the size and location of the perforation, how fast it is identified and repaired, the ability to seal the perforation, the chance of new attachment formation, the ability to clean and obturate the rest of the canal system, the presence of an associated periodontal pocket and microbial infection.

Root Fractures

As well as pain/tenderness on mastication, a sinus tract near the gingival margin or narrow deep periodontal pocket in an abhorrent position such as the buccal or palatal/lingual aspect may be the give away sign of a root fracture (Fig. 8.13). Radiographically, this may appear as a widening of the periodontal ligament, a lateral radiolucency or thin halo like apical radiolucency, however, to be seen radiographically the fracture must be parallel to the x-ray beam. The presence of a fracture with gingival sulcus/pocket involvement may mean a hopeless prognosis due to the bacterial invasion of the fracture space from the oral environment.

Root fractures may be diagnosed with a sharp probe, transillumination, dyes and magnification, parallax radiography depending on the position of the fracture in relation to the radiation beam and use of Tooth Slooth or FractFinder. Root fractures may also be discovered during surgical periodontal treatment and may often render the tooth unrestorable, as the fracture cannot be sealed.

Teeth with vertical fractures are of hopeless prognosis, as it would not be possible to seal this site of microbial ingress, and will eventually require extraction. It may be possible to palliatively manage associated pockets with root surface debridement and good oral hygiene. Horizontal fractures may be amenable to root canal treatment (Case 4), especially where a periodontal pocket has not yet formed.

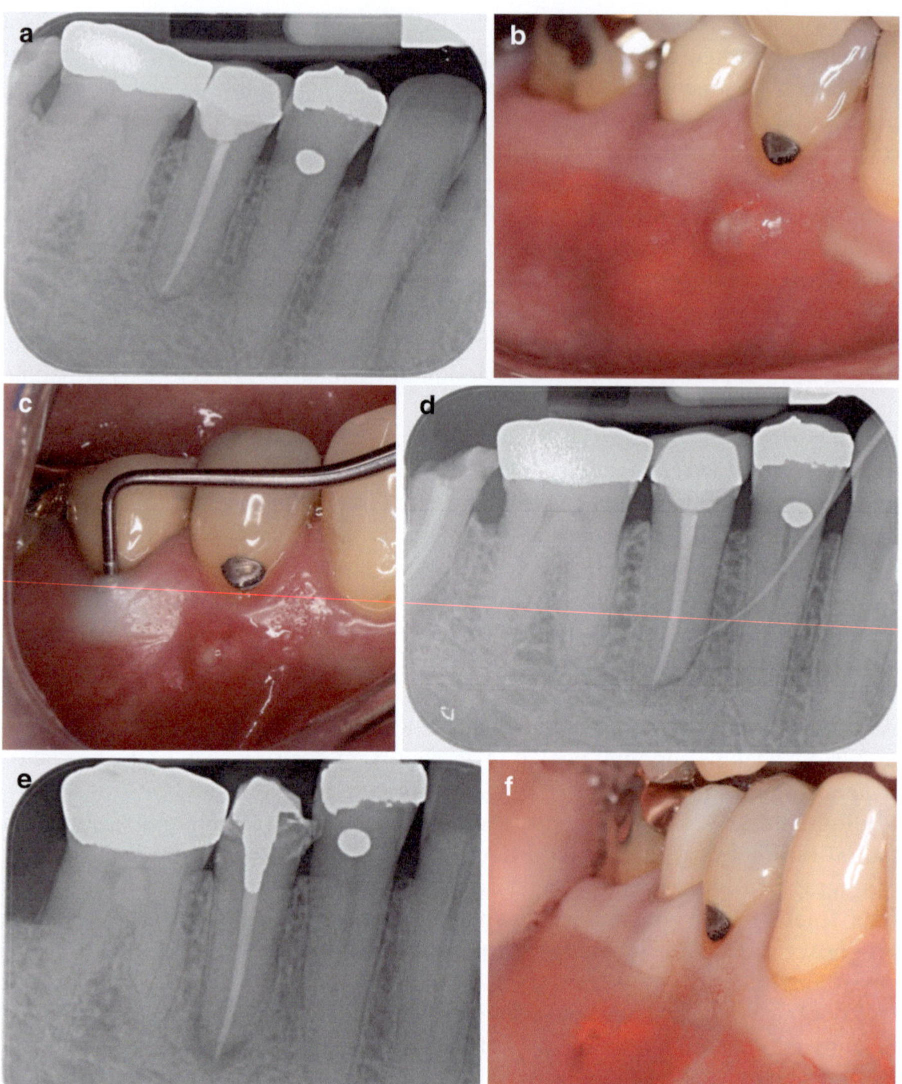

Fig. 8.13 Intra-oral photographs and LCPA radiographs of the LR5: Root fractures may present themselves as a lateral periodontal abscess, as in this example of the LR5 (**a** & **b**). Careful examination and special tests reveal the cause to be the LR5 (**c** & **d**). There may be little radiographic evidence of apical periodontitis as there is drainage through the single deep periodontal pocket and the buccally draining sinus. It is possible that there is a fracture present within the LR5. During root canal treatment, a fracture line was visible buccally, however as patency was achieved with consistent apex locator zero readings, and the periodontal pocket healed with instigation of root canal treatment and periodontal debridement under local anaesthesia, the fracture was accepted and the root canal treatment completed. Following completion of endodontic treatment, the buccally draining sinus resolved (**e** & **f**)

Root Resorption

Several types of resorption have been described earlier in this book. Replacement resorption is due to the inability of the connective tissue to form an attachment to denuded root dentine, however if less than 20% of the root surface is involved, it is possible to reverse the process of ankylosis. As the normal remodeling process of bone then replaces the tooth, the rate at which this occurs will depend on the patients' metabolic rate. Resorption may occur with long standing lesions or damage to cementum. Clinically these teeth give a 'metallic' sound on percussion with an absence of physiological movement. Radiographically, it will be difficult to visualise the periodontal ligament and may reveal a 'moth eaten' appearance around the root (Rotstein and Simon 2004). Depending on the position, resorption may be difficult to visualise with plain film radiographs, however, is visible on CBCT allowing differentiation between external and internal resorption. Apical root resorption is also possible with long-standing chronic infections such as untreated periodontal and endodontic disease, as seen in Fig. 8.14.

External cervical root resorption often is clinically asymptomatic and mostly detected radiographically (Rotstein and Simon 2004). Clinically, resorption is hard to probing and can be differentiated from soft caries. If located coronally and is undermining enamel, resorption often appears a pinkish hue with irregular enamel. Radiographically, either a well-circumscribed or irregular 'mottled' appearance is seen, with the outline of the root canal visible within the lesion, as the lesion often spreads laterally without invading the pulp. The radiopacity separating the root canal system is present because the pulp remains protected by a thin layer of pre-dentine (Rotstein and Simon 2004). Cervical resorption is most likely to present with periodontal pocketing (usually with a horizontal component), and trauma, orthodontic treatment or bleaching may have instigated it. There is usually good plaque control, yet gingival inflammation and bleeding. The granulation tissue bleeds on probing and there may be an associated periodontal abscess. Surgical treatment is required and this treatment may lead to necrosis of the pulp.

Internal resorption may present with signs of irreversible pulpitis, but also as a non-vital tooth with or without apical periodontitis (Cases 19 and 20). It is usually diagnosed from a radiograph, however in some occasions may be difficult to differentiate from external resorption (Case 21).

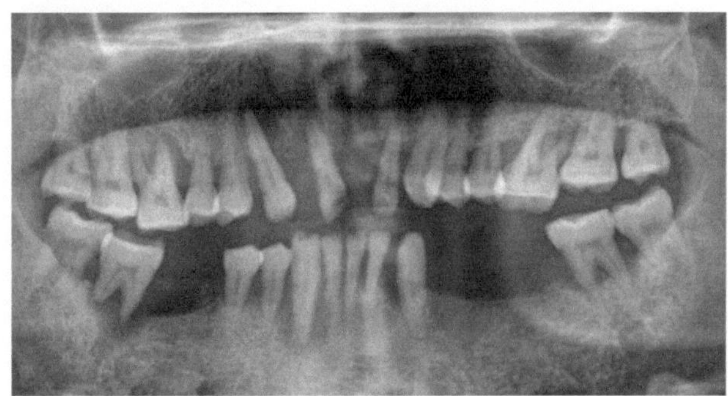

Fig. 8.14 DPT showing untreated periodontal disease has led to apical root resorption of the LR6

Case 19 A 56-year-old male patient presented with food packing between the LL67. This has been present for some time and developed into a dull aching pain when food trapping occurred. Clinically, no deep periodontal pockets were present, cavitation of the mesial aspect of the LL7 was not felt and none of the teeth were tender to percussion. There was no associated swelling, sinus or tenderness. An incidental finding on the radiographs was a resorptive defect on the mesial aspect of the LL7, with a possible cavitation visible mesially (Fig. 8.15a, b). The LL7 gave no response to sensibility testing. Is this internal or external resorption? What is the prognosis? Is it worth starting treatment?

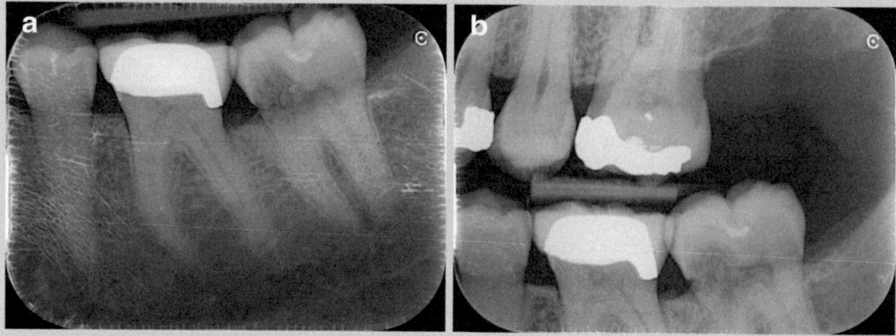

Fig. 8.15 (**a**) LCPA radiograph of the LL7 and (**b**) bitewing radiograph of the left side, both showing a radiolucency within the LL6

Case 20 A 42-year-old male presented, having 12-months previously suffered throbbing aching pain from the LL6. Clinical examination revealed no periodontal pockets, tenderness of the mesiobuccal cusp of the LL6 to percussion, no swelling, sinus or soft tissue tenderness (Fig. 8.16a, b). The LL6 and LL7 tested positively to electric pulp testing with lingering pain. The LL6 responded to cold testing, but the LL7 did not. The LL7 was not tender to percussion. No symptoms were elicited with a Tooth Slooth. Radiographic examination revealed furcal resorption of the LL6, which may have been external or internal in origin (Fig. 8.17a–e). What are the options for such a tooth and the potential sequelae? Is it worth starting treatment?

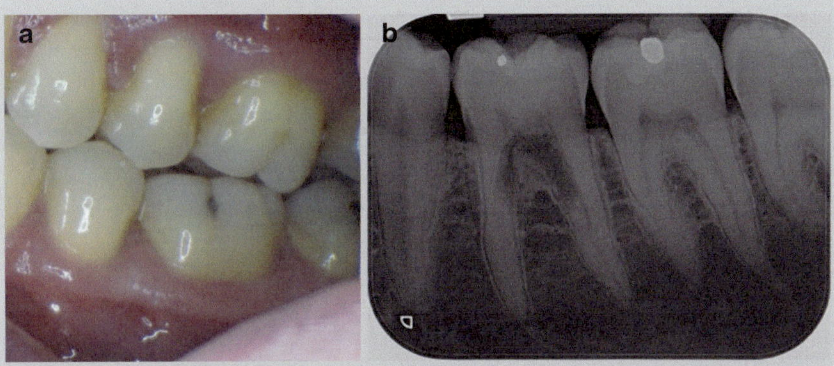

Fig. 8.16 (**a**) Photograph of the left side showing a minimally restored LL6 without any sign of gingival inflammation. (**b**) LCPA radiograph of the LL6 showing resorption of the furcal aspect of the LL6

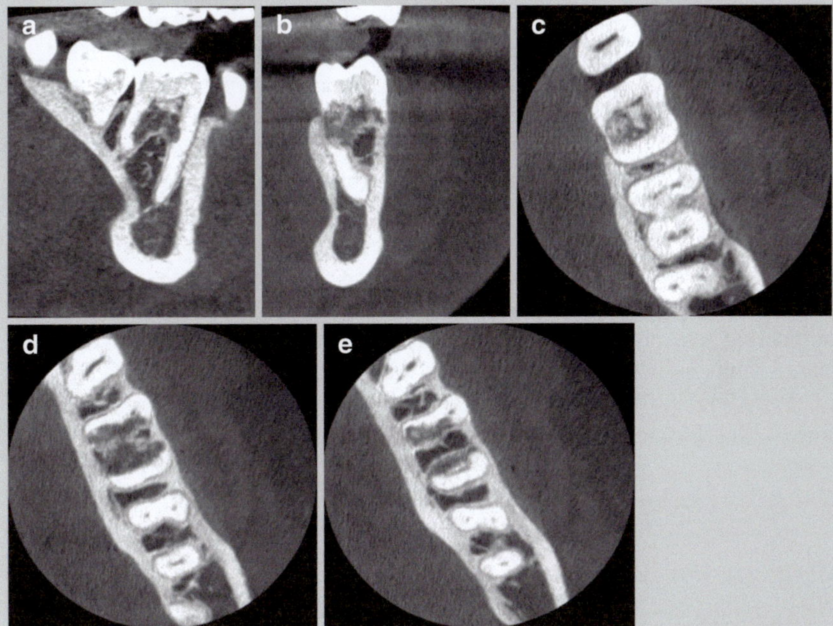

Fig. 8.17 (**a**) Sagittal CBCT image of the LL6. (**b**) Coronal CBCT image of the LL6. (**c–e**) Axial CBCT images of the LL6

Case 21 A 32-year-old patient presented in with buccal swelling and sinus within the attached gingivae adjacent to the UL12 (Fig. 8.18a, b). There was a history of trauma to the UL12 at age 6 years and endodontic treatment had been provided during childhood. At presentation, deep periodontal pockets were not seen. The patient then presented 6 months later for endodontic re-treatment of the UL12, at which point, a 10 mm pocket was seen at the mesial line angle, with bleeding on probing and suppuration. During this treatment, the periodontal pocket was also debrided with ultrasonic scaling. At the second endodontic treatment appointment, a month later, the periodontal pocket had reduced to 8 mm, with slight bleeding on probing and no suppuration. The pocket also appeared narrower and the patient was no longer able to insert a narrow interdental brush vertically in the pocket. The UL2 was obturated with gutta percha and the UL1 was obturated with MTA followed by gutta percha (Fig. 8.19a). During endodontic treatment of the UL1, external resorption of almost the entire buccal wall of the coronal half of the root was seen. At the 3 month review, although the buccal swelling and sinus had resolved, and the periodontal pocket had reduced to 5 mm, there was still a small amount of bleeding on probing with suppuration. The patient reported daily draining of pus from the gingival crevice. The UL1 was a grey discolouration and the mobility (grade I) had not improved. No further improvement was expected due to the labial wall of the root of the UL1 being almost completely resorbed. The patient opted for extraction of the UL1 and replacement with an immediate denture, followed by a resin-retained bridge using the UR1 as an abutment. The presence and extent of the resorptive lesion is not visible from the initial radiograph taken in January 2021 (Fig. 8.19a). However the post-operative radiograph was at a different angle revealing the resorptive defect (Fig. 8.19b). It is difficult to know if this was initially internal or external resorption. When the patient presented for review of the UL2, the buccal sinus associated with the UL1 was still present, although reduced. A LCPA radiograph of the UL1 revealed part of the root had been left behind (Fig. 8.19c). Extraction of this allowed for complete healing (Fig. 8.19d).

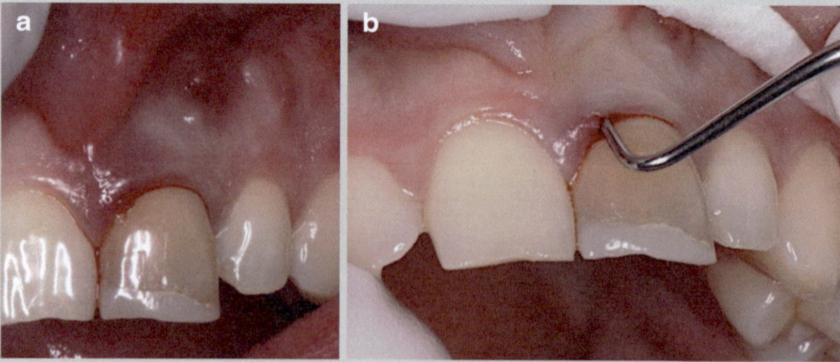

Fig. 8.18 (**a**) Photograph of the UL1 revealing a buccal sinus in attached gingivae between the UL12. (**b**) Photograph of the UL1 showing deep periodontal pocketing associated with the mesial line angle of the UL1

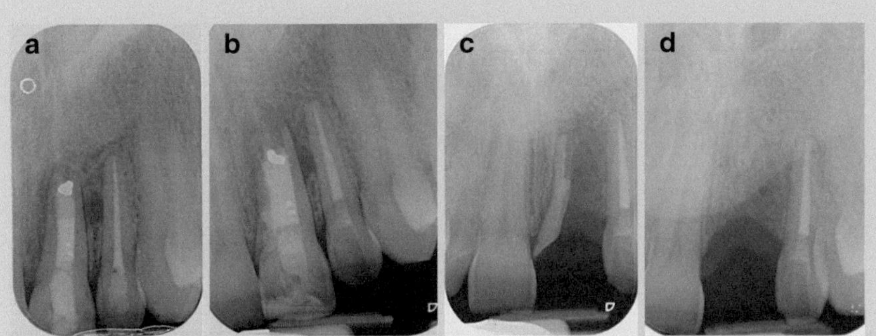

Fig. 8.19 (**a**) Pre-operative LCPA radiograph of the UL12 (Jan 2021). (**b**) Post-operative LCPA radiograph of the UL12 following endodontic re-treatment (Jul 2021). (**c**) LCPA radiograph of the UL1 space where part of the root of the UL1 had been left behind (Jan 2022). (**d**) LCPA radiograph of the UL12 space showed complete healing (Aug 2022)

If there is a primary endodontic cause, root canal treatment alone will resolve the lesion. If an endodontic lesion causes the periodontal pocket and there is a long-standing pocket, theoretically it is possible to develop calculus in the pocket that requires periodontal debridement also (Case 22). If a separate periodontal pocket is present and stable without an active lesion, active periodontal treatment is not required, however, supportive periodontal care is recommended, especially for those pockets that are 5 mm of deeper. When the status of the periodontal tissues at the time of non-surgical endodontic treatment was considered, the survival of endodontically treated teeth in periodontally sound patients has been shown to be 90% at 9 years with that for teeth with 'mild' periodontitis being 71% and that for teeth with 'moderate' periodontitis being 59% (Khalighinejad et al. 2017). Better survival (85%) was seen for endodontically treated teeth where patients engaged in supportive periodontal therapy when compared to survival rates (61%) for those who failed to comply with supportive periodontal care, and smokers were at higher risk of failure of endodontically treated teeth (Khalighinejad et al. 2017).

Case 22 The UR45 were endodontically treated following trauma in 2010 (Fig. 8.20a). Due to the shape of the roots, and possibly as a result of the initial trauma, a pre-operative pocket depth of 8 mm was present on the distal aspect of the UR4 and mesial aspect of the UR5. In 2022 (Fig. 8.20b) these pockets had reduced to 5 mm on the distopalatal and mesial aspect of the UR4. The patient's diligent oral hygiene regime had also led to buccal cervical wear cavities (Fig. 8.21a). Following oral health education, root surface debridement and restoration of the cervical wear cavities (Fig. 8.21b) resulted in reduction of the periodontal pockets to 3 mm on the distopalatal aspect of the UR4, and the mesiopalatal aspect of the UR5, and 2 mm on the buccal aspect of these teeth, with recession of between 5 and 8 mm. It is possible that there is a separated instrument in the distobuccal root, and the mesiobuccal root may not be ideally filled in the three-rooted UR4. This could be a perio-endo lesion managed well with periodontal and endodontic treatment, in a patient committed to optimal oral hygiene.

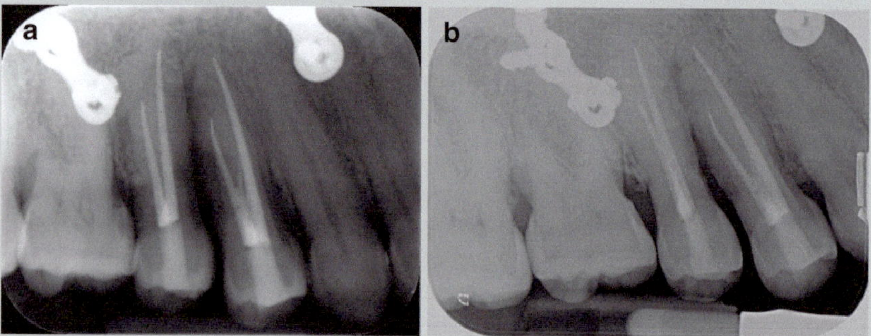

Fig. 8.20 (**a**) LCPA radiograph of the UR45 (2010) following root canal treatment. (**b**) LCPA radiograph of the UR45 after 12 years (2022)

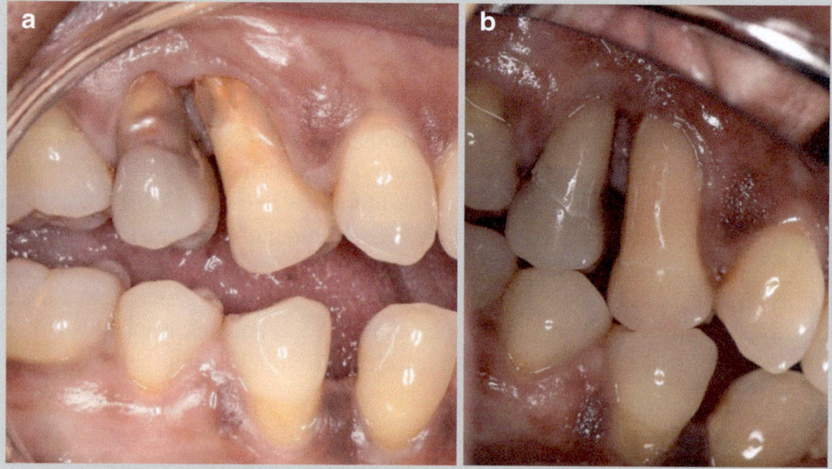

Fig. 8.21 (**a**) Photograph of the UR45 showing buccal recession almost exposing the root canal filling. (**b**) Photograph of the UR45 following restoration to avoid further wear of the roots

Endodontic disease should be managed with endodontic treatment/re-treatment, under rubber dam using sodium hypochlorite and EDTA as irrigants, using an appropriate intracanal medication between visits, aiming to achieve a root filling without voids, to within 2 mm of the radiographic apex. The preparation and taper should allow for sufficient irrigant to reach the apex. This should lead to healing

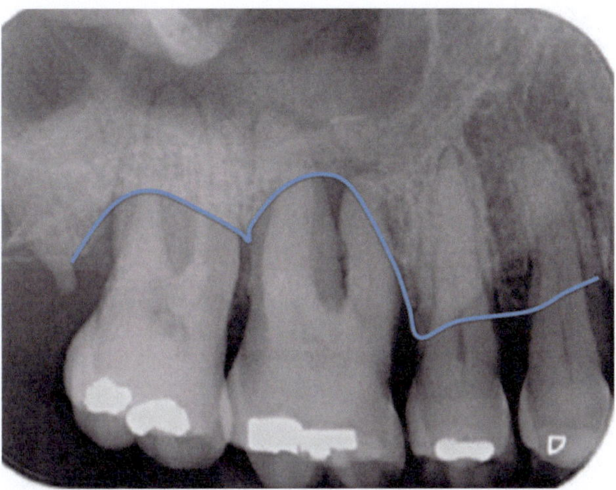

Fig. 8.22 LCPA radiograph of the UR4567. In a case such as this UR6, despite periodontal and endodontic treatment, it is unlikely that the furcation bone loss will fill in. The best one can expect without surgical intervention is bony infill to the level of the horizontal bone loss (blue line)

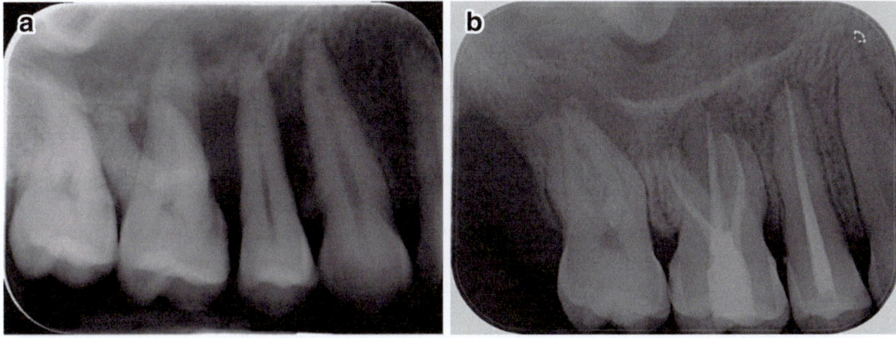

Fig. 8.23 LCPA radiographs of the UR56. A patient presented with apical radiolucencies associated with the UR567. Radiographically it appeared as though there was periodontal breakdown and possible perio-endo lesions were diagnosed (**a**). These teeth were unrestored, non-responsive to sensibility testing and yet, without periodontal pocketing or mobility. Endodontic treatment led to complete healing and bony infill (**b**). The UR7 is also planned for endodontic treatment (radiographs courtesy of Mr. Nalin Dhamecha)

and resolution of draining sinuses, either through the periodontal pocket or adjacent to it. There should be bony infill as seen radiographically (Figs. 8.22 and 8.23a, b). In the absence of healing, endodontic surgery may be required. Annual clinical and radiographic review until healing has occurred is recommended. If the periodontal component does not heal with this treatment, periodontal treatment may also be required. It should be noted that both periodontal and endodontic infections might recur, and require additional treatment, therefore, regular review and early intervention is essential. Left untreated, they may lead to perio-endo lesions of poor prognosis.

References

Abbott RV. Classification, diagnosis and clinical manifestations of apical periodontitis. Endo Topics. 2004;8(1):36–54.

Abbott PV, Salgado JC. Strategies for the endodontic management of concurrent endodontic and periodontal diseases. Aust Dent J. 2009;54:S70–85.

Basten CH-J, Ammons WF Jr, Persson R. Long-term evaluation of root resected molars: a retrospective study. Int J Periodontics Restorative Dent. 1996;16:206.

Blomlof LB. Relationship between periapical and periodontal status. J Clin Periodontol. 1993;20:117–23.

Blomlöf L, Lindskog S, Hammarstrom L. Influence of pulpal treatments on cell and tissue reactions in the marginal periodontium. J Periodontol. 1988;59:577–83.

Chapple ILC, Lumley PJ. The perio-endo interface. Dent Update. 1999;26:331–41.

Christie WH, Holthuis AF. The endo-perio problem in dental practice: diagnosis and prognosis. J Can Dent Assoc. 1990;56(11):1005–11.

Clauder T, Shin SJ. Repair of perforations with MTA: clinical actions and mechanisms of action. Endod Topics. 2009;15:32–55.

Czarnecki RT, Schilder H. A histological evaluation of the human pulp in teeth with varying degrees of periodontal disease. J Endod. 1979;5(8):242–52.

Diem CR, Bower GM, Ferrigno PD, Fedi PF Jr. Regeneration of the attachment apparatus on pulpless teeth denuded on cementum in Rhesus monkey. J Periodontol. 1974;45:18.

Ehnevid H, Jansson L, Lindskog S, Blomlof L. Periodontal healing in teeth with periapical lesions. A clinical retrospective study. J Clin Periodontol. 1993;20:254–8.

Farzaneh M, Abitbol S, Friedman S. Treatment outcome in endodontics: the Toronto study. Phases I and II: orthograde retreatment. J Endod. 2004;30(9):627–33.

Ford TR, Torabinejad M, McKendry DJ, Hong CU, Kariyawasam SP. Use of mineral trioxide aggregate for repair of furcal perforations. Oral Surg Oral Med Oral Pathol Oral Radiol Endod. 1995;79(6):756–63.

Fuss Z, Trope M. Root perforations: classification and treatment choices based on prognostic factors. Endod Dent Traumatol. 1996;12(6):255–64.

Hargreaves KM, Cohen S, Berman LH. Cohen's pathways of the pulp. 10th ed. St. Louis: Mosby Elsevier; 2011.

Harrington GW. The perio-endo question: differential diagnosis. Dent Clin N Am. 1979;23:673–69.

Jansson LE, Ehnevid H. The influence of endodontic infection on periodontal status in mandibular molars. J Periodontol. 1998;69:1392–6.

Jansson L, Ehnevid H, Lindskog S, Blomlof L. Relationship between periapical and periodontal status. A clinical retrospective study. J Clin Periodontol. 1993;20:117–23.

Khalighinejad N, Aminoshariae A, Kulild JC, Wang J, Mickel A. The influence of periodontal status on endodontically treated teeth: 9-year survival analysis. J Endod. 2017;43(11):1781–5.

Naik RM, Pudakalkatti PS, Hattarki SA. Can MTA be: miracle trioxide aggregate? J Indian Soc Periodontol. 2014;18(1):5–8.

Nair PNR. Apical periodontitis: a dynamic encounter between root canal infection and host response. Periodontology. 1997;13:121–48.

Nair PNR. On the causes of persistent apical periodontitis: a review. Int Endod J. 2006;39:249–81.

Nair PNR, Pajarola G, Schroeder HE. Types and incidence of human periapical lesions obtained with extracted teeth. Oral Surg Oral Med Oral Pathol Oral Radiol Endod. 1996;81:93–102.

Ng YL, Mann V, Gulabivala K. A prospective study of the factors affecting outcomes of nonsurgical root canal treatment: part 1: periapical health. Int Endod J. 2011;44(7):583–609.

Nicholls E. Treatment of traumatic perforations of the pulp cavity. Oral Surg Oral Med Oral Pathol. 1962;15:603–12.

Parirokh M, Torabinejad M, Dummer PMH. Mineral trioxide aggregate and other bioactive endodontic cements: an updated overview – part I: vital pulp therapy. Int Endod J. 2018;51:177–205.

Perlmutter S, Tagger M, Tagger E, Abram M. Effect of the endodontic status of the tooth on experimental periodontal re-attachment in baboons: a preliminary investigation. Oral Surg Oral Med Oral Pathol. 1987;63:232.

Ramfjord SP, Ash MM. Periodontology and periodontics. Philadelphia: Saunders; 1979. p. 247–309.

Ricucci D, Langeland K. Apical limit of root canal instrumentation and obturation, part 2. A histological study. Int Endod J. 1998;31(6):394–409.

Rotstein I, Simon JH. Diagnosis, prognosis and decision-making in the treatment of combined periodontal-endodontic lesions. Periodontol. 2004;34:165–203.

Sanders JJ, Sepe WW, Bowers GM, Koch RW, Williams JE, Lekas JS, Mellonig JT, Pelleu GB Jr, Gambill V. Clinical evaluation of freeze-dried bone allografts in periodontal osseous defects. Part III. Composite freeze-dried bone allografts with and without autogenous bone grafts. J Periodontol. 1983;54(1):1–8.

Solomon C, Chalfin H, Kellert M, Weseley P. The endodontic-periodontal lesion: a rational approach to treatment. J Am Dent Assoc. 1995;126(4):473–9.

Strömberg T, Hasselgren G, Bergstedt H. Endodontic treatment of traumatic root perforations in man. A clinical and roentgenological follow-up study. Sven Tandlak Tidskr. 1972;65(9):457–466.

Torabinejad M, Watson TF, Pitt Ford TR. Sealing ability of a mineral trioxide aggregate when used as a root end filling material. J Endod. 1993;19(12):591–5.

Torabinejad M, Parirokh M, Dummer PMH. Mineral trioxide aggregate and other bioactive endodontic cements: an updated overview – part II: other clinical applications and complications. Int Endod J. 2018;51:284–317.

World Health Organisation. Application of the International Classification of Diseases to dentistry and stomatology. 3rd ed. Geneva: WHO; 1995. p. 66–7.

Zehnder M, Gold SI, Hasselgren G. Pathologic interaction in pulpal and periodontal tissues. J Clin Periodontol. 2002;29:663–71.

True Perio-Endo Lesions

9

Abstract

This chapter discusses true Perio-Endo lesions, the diagnosis and management of them, as well as the expected outcomes of treatment.

True Perio-Endo Lesions

Perio-endo lesions are as a result of the two soft tissue lesions, periodontal and endodontic, merging (Fig. 9.1). They may present with a periodontal pocket, pain, swelling, suppuration and increased tooth mobility. Although, a single periodontal pocket may also indicate iatrogenic root perforation, vertical root fracture or external root resorption. It may be difficult to diagnose whether the origin was periodontal or endodontic, and it may be difficult to know if the lesion is being maintained by plaque or root canal infection. Pulp death may have occurred due to periodontal disease or developed independently. The pathogenesis of the true combined lesions resemble pathogenesis of endodontic lesions and periodontal lesions, which eventually merge, and cannot be distinguished from those of primary endodontic origin with secondary periodontal involvement and those of primary periodontal origin with secondary endodontic involvement (Anand et al. 2012a).

The prognosis of true perio-endo lesions may be guarded or poor as the bacterial biofilm on the root surface may no longer be accessible with non-surgical periodontal or endodontic treatment. If a portion of the lesion is sustained by the root canal infection independent of the periodontal disease, the potential for the periodontal tissues to regenerate is much increased with endodontic treatment, and in these cases there may be an option to perform root canal treatment and delay the periodontal

S. Eliyas, *The Periodontic-Endodontic Interface*,
https://doi.org/10.1007/978-3-031-49937-1_9

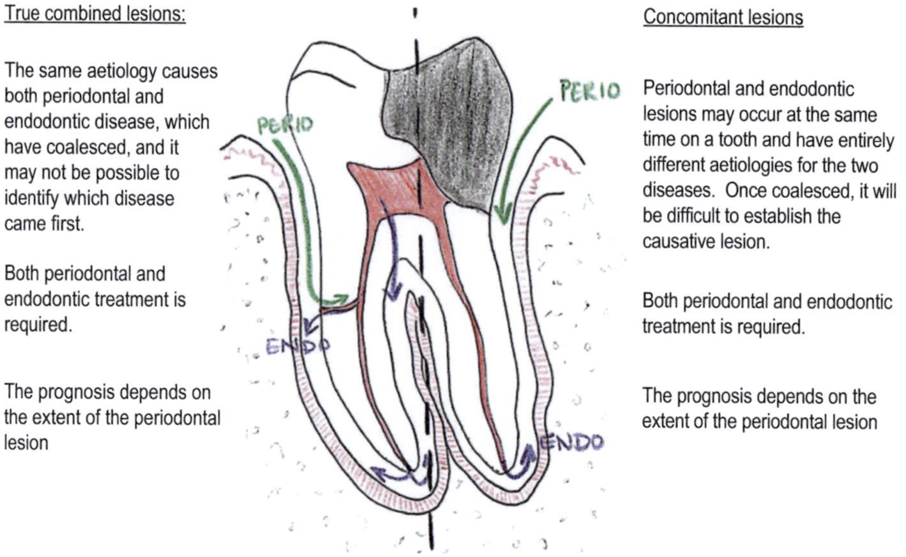

Fig. 9.1 Perio-endo lesions, some concomitant and others truly combined

treatment until the outcome can be evaluated. In most cases though, if there were a periodontal pocket present, it would be sensible to also root surface debride the pocket at the time of endodontic treatment as the tooth is already anaesthetised, for the periodontal biofilm to also be disturbed. Endodontic re-treatment should be considered an adjunct to periodontal treatment when a root canal filling is defective or shows signs of being associated with increased pocket depths, more marginal bone loss and retarded/impaired periodontal tissue healing subsequent to periodontal treatment (Jansson et al. 1993; Ehnevid et al. 1993). In 'mild' cases of periodontal disease the presence or absence of root canal treatment or infections have been seen to make no difference to the periodontal outcome (Miyashita et al. 1998). Teeth with endodontic treatment and periodontal disease may have a poorer outcome than teeth with periodontal disease and healthy pulps (Jaoui et al. 1995). After treatment, the periodontium heals not with junctional epithelium adjacent to cementum, however, with a long junctional epithelium adjacent to dentine (Lindskog et al. 1993). Therefore, care should be taken when providing root surface debridement as not to remove the cementum.

Although the microbial species are similar in endodontic lesions and periodontal lesions, the microbial load and number of species may be different. The microbial biofilm may be more complex as a result in perio-endo lesions (Kobayashi et al. 1990; Trope et al. 1992; Sundqvist 1992; Kurihara et al. 1995). The microbes from the periodontal lesion and endodontic lesion may cross seed (Kipioti et al. 1984; Dongari and Lambrianidis 1988; Kerekes and Olsen 1990) and it may not be possible to achieve an apical seal as the periodontal lesion may feed the bacteria within accessory canals in the apical third of the root. In perio-endo lesions of periodontal origin, immunological and microbiological study suggests the source of endodontic infection is the periodontal pocket bacteria (Kurihara et al. 1995).

Lateral periodontal cysts may also present this way, with gingival swelling, with or without pain/pain on palpation. Radiographic examination will reveal a well-circumscribed oval or round lesion with sclerotic margins. Histopathological analysis will show the presence of an epithelium or epithelium like lining. This is a slow growing lesion that does not resolve with periodontal or endodontic treatment (Odell and Cawson 2017). Scleroderma, metastatic carcinoma and osteosarcoma can mimic perio-endo lesions, however, these will not resolve with endodontic and periodontal treatment.

The Diagnosis of True Perio-Endo Lesions

The diagnosis of true perio-endo lesions, and differentiation from both periodontal disease with endodontic manifestations and endodontic disease with periodontal manifestations is difficult (Case 23). Signs and symptoms of both diseases are present with symptoms of bad taste, draining pus from gingival crevice, deep periodontal pockets, tenderness to percussion, and irregular results to sensibility testing. If the tooth is vital, this excludes an endodontic cause and needs periodontal treatment, and if the tooth is non-vital, there may be an endodontic contribution to the lesion. Sometimes, radiographs can allude to a perio-endo lesion with 'halo' and 'j-shaped' radiolucencies, and surgical exploration can find no communication with the apex, or find other reasons for pathology such as cracks or fractures.

Case 23 This LR6 was grade 2 mobile, not tender to percussion and presented with a 8 mm pocket on the distal aspect. On first glance at the radiograph, it may appear as though the LR6 was mobile as a result of almost 50% horizontal bone loss (Fig. 9.2). However, a similar level of bone loss was present on the single rooted LR5, and yet this tooth was not mobile. There must be another reason for the mobility. The LR6 was not occlusally overloaded, therefore, there must be some apical pathology contributing to the mobility. The LR6 was found to give a negative response to sensibility testing (by placing a probe on tooth structure, and connecting the electric pulp tester to the probe). This may be a true perio-endo lesion, where the LR6 lost vitality as a result of crown preparation, and concomitantly was periodontally involved, and the two lesions combined distally. What percentage of teeth lose vitality once prepared for a crown? Why is a frank apical area associated with the LR6 not visible?

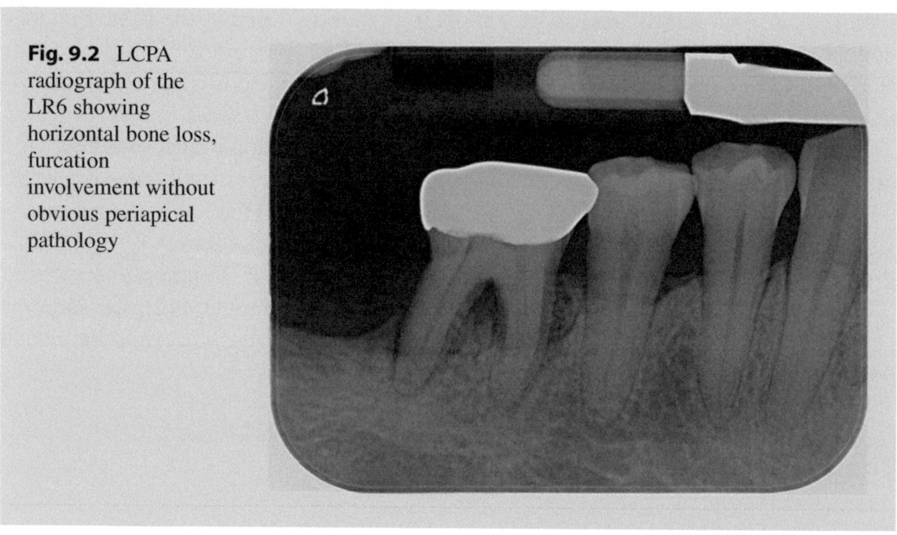

Fig. 9.2 LCPA radiograph of the LR6 showing horizontal bone loss, furcation involvement without obvious periapical pathology

The Management and Outcomes of True Perio-Endo Lesions

When considering treatment, the prognosis of the tooth and strategic value must be considered first, as well as the possibility of providing predictable high quality treatment that is likely to improve the life of the tooth. From a periodontal point of view, the ability of the patient to be able to access difficult root anatomy and be able to maintain optimal oral hygiene will determine the outcome. Complex intervention is not appropriate if the patient is unable to prevent daily plaque accumulation, unless treatment is also going to lead to alteration of the anatomy to improve access to such areas.

In a perio-endo lesion, healing following one aspect (either periodontal or endodontic), may lead to reconsidering the diagnosis of a combined perio-endo lesion. Some have suggested that endodontic treatment ought to be provided first, as this can lead to healing and confirmation of a diagnosis (Schmidt et al. 2014; Anand et al. 2012b; Abbott and Salgado 2009; Chapple and Lumley 1999). In a lesion likely to be combined, periodontal treatment alone does not often lead to healing. If after localised periodontal debridement, suppuration remains, then pulpal necrosis ought to be suspected before pursuing periodontal surgery (Anand et al. 2012b). This discussion of whether root canal treatment or periodontal treatment should be carried out first and the time frame for review before instigating further treatment has been ongoing (Schmidt et al. 2014).

Essentially, a primary endodontic lesion with secondary periodontal manifestations will heal with endodontic treatment alone, and should be reviewed at 3 months after endodontic treatment. Primary periodontal lesions with secondary manifestations of endodontic disease and true perio-endo lesion will require both periodontal and endodontic treatment, however, the order in which this is provided may vary.

There are a number of treatment strategies available (Abbott and Salgado 2009; Chapple and Lumley 1999; Zehnder et al. 2002):

(a) Initial endodontic treatment, dressing of the tooth with a medicament and then providing periodontal treatment, before completing endodontic treatment
(b) Initial periodontal treatment and then endodontic treatment
(c) Simultaneous endodontic and periodontal treatment

Option (a) and (b) may be necessary when separate periodontal and endodontic specialists are treating the patient, as combined treatment may be more difficult to achieve logistically. However, when the tooth is anaesthetised for endodontic treatment, it is an opportunity to also provide root surface debridement.

Treatment of Concurrent Endodontic and Periodontal Lesions without Communication

When periodontal pathology and either irreversible pulpitis or necrosis of the pulp is present, both root canal treatment and periodontal treatment will be required. It is advisable to obturate the canal system as soon as possible and provide periodontal treatment at the same visit. The prognosis will be better if the two lesions do not communicate (Abbott 1998), but ultimately will be determined by the outcome of the periodontal treatment and the patient's ability to maintain optimal oral hygiene (Anand et al. 2012b; Jansson et al. 1995). It is thought that endodontic infections could stimulate downgrowth of epithelium along denuded dentine with marginal communication, leading to more bone loss (Abbott and Salgado 2009; Abbott 1998; Blomlöf et al. 1988). Some have suggested a three-fold increase in the rate of marginal bone loss in periodontally susceptible patients when there is ongoing infection of the root canal system and periapical pathology (Jansson et al. 1995).

Concurrent endodontic and periodontal disease without communication should ideally be both endodontically and periodontally treated from the beginning. However, if the patient presents with an acute exacerbation, it may be more suitable to immediately treat either the acute apical abscess (with endodontic treatment) or the acute periodontal abscess (with periodontal treatment) to bring the patient back to comfort. If the patient is symptomatic, it may be advisable to carry out non-surgical endodontic treatment prior to periodontal treatment. All restorations provided should be with good margins to seal the endodontic treatment, but also, not to have overhangs that may complicate periodontal treatment. The presence of microbes within the canal during periodontal treatment may mean the possibility of microbes and their toxins escaping through dentinal tubules (exposed if cementum is disturbed during periodontal treatment) into the periodontal tissues, which may delay periodontal healing or lead to external inflammatory root resorption.

The timing of endodontic and periodontal treatment in the management of perio-endo lesions without communication has been previously considered. When periodontal treatment and endodontic treatment were performed simultaneously for perio-endo lesions, and compared with periodontal treatment 3 months after completion of endodontic treatment, the periodontal healing was comparable in both groups (Gupta et al. 2015).

Treatment of Concurrent Endodontic and Periodontal Lesions with Communication

Concurrent endodontic and periodontal disease with communication should ideally be both endodontically and periodontally treated in parallel. Some have recommended that the tooth is still endodontically treated initially, dressed with Ledermix to control symptoms first, then after 4 weeks, dressed with a 50:50 mixture of Ledermix and Calcium Hydroxide. Following this, periodontal treatment is to be commenced, which will include improvement in oral hygiene and root surface debridement, and may include surgical treatment such as open flap debridement. Three months later, the periodontal status should be reassessed, and if the periodontal tissues are healing, the final obturation of the canal system and coronal seal can be provided. If there is no healing, re-dressing of the tooth with a mixture of Ledermix and Calcium hydroxide and further periodontal treatment, which may be surgical or non-surgical is recommended (Abbott and Salgado 2009). The reason for non-healing should also be considered, such as the presence of a crack, poor oral hygiene and difficult anatomy leading to poor oral hygiene. Surgical intervention, such as root amputation or hemisection, may be required. If the periodontal prognosis is poor, the tooth may require extraction. Once there are signs of periodontal healing, the root canal treatment can be completed and a satisfactory coronal seal provided, followed by regular periodontal re-assessment. Delaying this stage may save the patient the cost of complex treatment for a tooth that does not heal (Abbott and Salgado 2009; Abbott 1998). For true combined lesions, Chapple and Lumley suggest root canal treatment, re-assessment clinically and radiographically at 2–3 months, periodontal treatment if there are no signs of resolution, followed by clinical and radiographic re-assessment at 2–3 months (Chapple and Lumley 1999). If both periodontal and endodontic components of the lesion are obvious, it may be of advantage to complete all treatment as soon as possible. Some protocols have included completion of non-surgical root canal treatment, assessment of healing 1 month later, and if a periodontal pocket of more than 5 mm is present, non-surgical root surface debridement under local anaesthesia, followed by re-assessment at 3 months (Vakalis et al. 2005).

Although endodontic treatment boasts outcomes of around 95%, these figures fall to around 78% when teeth with perio-endo lesions are studied (Kim et al. 2008; Song et al. 2018). In some cases, survival at 5 years has been reported around 60% (Schacher et al. 2007). In another study by Fang et al. (2021), a fairly large population of patients with combined perio-endo lesions, half were provided with root canal treatment only, and the other half were treated with non-surgical endodontic and periodontal treatment. Outcomes in terms of periodontal indices, reduction in inflammatory markers, symptoms and tooth retention were better in the group that received both periodontal and endodontic treatment (Fang et al. 2021). When the timing of each modality of treatment were considered for perio-endo lesions with communication, there are few high quality studies, and what is available, has recommended either endodontic intervention prior to or simultaneously with periodontal treatment (Friedrich et al. 2023).

Regenerative Techniques

Although, it was always thought that teeth with true combined lesions will have a poor prognosis (Whyman 1988), recent advances in regeneration have saved teeth of hopeless prognosis (Cortellini et al. 2011; Cortellini et al. 2020). In generalised chronic periodontitis patients (stage III or IV), successful regeneration of 'hopeless' teeth, i.e. those with a single tooth with perio-endo involvement and bone loss to the apex has been demonstrated (Cortellini et al. 2011, 2020). In these cases, the patients underwent non-surgical periodontal treatment; root canal treatment or re-treatment, and hyper-mobile teeth were splinted to adjacent teeth pre-surgery. Surgical regeneration included a papilla preservation flap, defect debridement, root planing including debridement of the apical area of the root with sonic diamond scalers and the placement of a variety of regenerative materials. Post-operative Doxycycline (100 mg) for 1 week and chlorhexidine mouthwash three times daily and 'weekly prophylaxis' without allowing the patient to brush, floss or chew in that area for 3–8 weeks was the protocol, after which full oral hygiene was resumed. The splints were removed after 1 year, with 5-year survival rates of 92% (Cortellini et al. 2011). With strict 3-monthly supportive periodontal care, 10-year survival rates were 88% (Cortellini et al. 2020). Endodontic surgery (i.e. resection of 3 mm of the root apex and provision of an apical seal) was not provided.

Guided tissue regeneration (GTR) prevents epithelial downgrowth and provides a scaffold for regeneration of periodontal architecture. Platelet-rich fibrin (PRF) has been used as a bioactive scaffold. Studies have started to evaluate the use of GTR and PRF in the management of vertical bone defects in teeth with perio-endo lesions (Rosen et al. 2023; Ustaoğlu et al. 2020). A systematic review included three randomised controlled trials and a prospective cohort study, and grouped together the results of 125 teeth in 125 patients over a follow up period of 12–60 months. Complete healing after surgical endodontic treatment using adjunctive GTR was reported to be 58% in teeth with perio-endo lesions (Rosen et al. 2023). Forty-five patients with residual two or three walled defects with deep pockets, after treatment with simultaneous non-surgical endodontic and full-mouth periodontal treatment, were treated with open flap debridement alone, GTR or PRF. Both GTR and PRF groups had better outcomes of periodontal healing and attachment gain than OFD alone. No significant difference was seen between the GTR and PRF groups (Ustaoğlu et al. 2020). Figure 9.3 shows that perio-endo

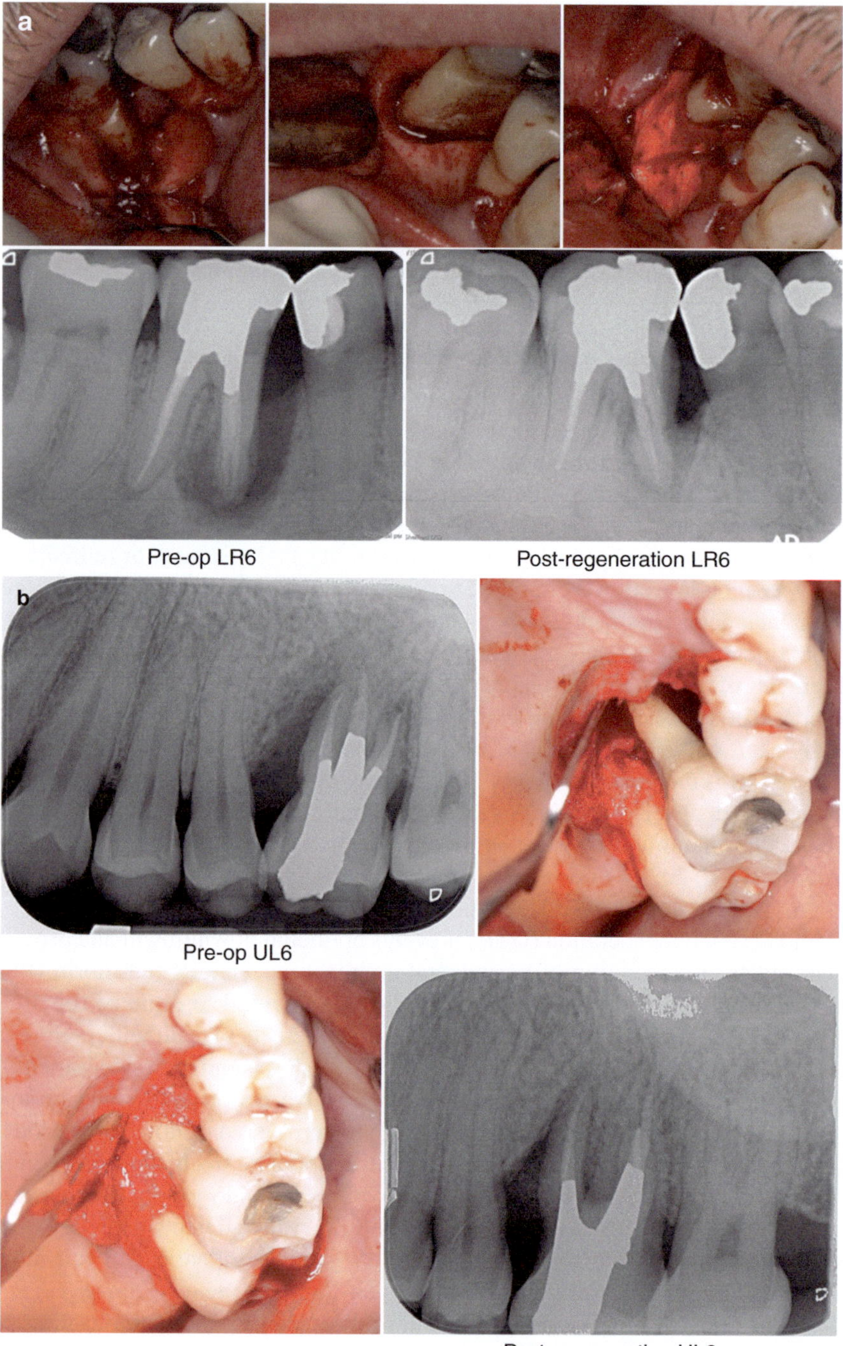

Fig. 9.3 Intra-oral photographs and radiographs of a LR6 (**a**) and UL6 (**b**), during and after regeneration with xenograft, with (**a**) and without (**b**) a membrane. Often granulation tissue needs removal to reveal the bony cavity that can be filled loosely with a scaffold to allow healing by regeneration

lesions with communication that have two or three walled defects are amenable to regenerative techniques.

Treatment with Root Resection/Hemisection/Root Amputation

Removal of a root is considered when one of the roots is of poor prognosis with a perio-endo lesion (or devoid of bone), where the other roots of a multi-rooted tooth have good bone support and better prognosis. For mandibular molars, removal of the mesial or distal roots may be termed hemisection or bicuspidisation and that for maxillary molars is termed root amputation (Khandelwal et al. 2020). Such treatment is only possible for teeth with divergent roots. Usually the indications are multi-rooted teeth with root fractures, perforations, root caries, dehiscence/fenestrations, external resorption involving one root, impaired endodontic treatment of a particular root (for example unable to gain patency or fractured instrument present), severe periodontal disease affecting only one root, and grade II or III furcations. Root amputation is not possible in fused roots and spindly remaining roots may be useless. Consider the occlusal forces, tooth restorability and the value of the remaining tooth (Case 24). It is likely that reshaping of the occlusal table is necessary, and restoration of the clinical crown in essential. The failure of these teeth is usually as a result of caries or failure of the endodontic treatment, if the periodontal status is stable. 10-year survival rates for rootresected molars have been reported to be between 62% and 96% (Langer et al. 1981; Carnevale et al. 1998; Bergenholtz 1972; Bühler 1988; Blomlöf et al. 1997; Carnevale et al. 1991; Park et al. 2009). Extractions have been reported to be due to endodontic failures, caries, periodontal disease progression and root fracture. When root resection was compared with implant survival, 15-year survival of 84–96.8% for resected roots and 96–97% for molar implants have been reported (Fugazzotto 2001; Kinsel et al. 1998).

Prior to resection/hemisection/amputation of roots, endodontic treatment should be completed first, with a good Nayyar core amalgam restoration to make polishing of the amputated root easier. Although composite restoration is possible, the sealing ability may be more difficult to predict. Sealing of the root stump after root resection is more difficult than polishing the existing restoration. When vital root amputation was performed, vitality was only maintained in 38% of teeth at 1 year and 13% of teeth at 5 years (Filipowicz et al. 1984), therefore, endodontic treatment before root resection is recommended. Root canal treatment after root resection may also be more difficult (in term of isolation and maintaining coronal seal from the root stump and sclerosis of the remaining pulp as a result of the insult). During emergency root canal treatment, it may be snesible to fill the canal with non-setting CaOH, however, this may require sealing during the root amputation surgery, which is technique sensitive. Ideally endodontic treatment for the other canals must be also performed, with well obturated and sealed coronal aspects, before the periodontal surgery (Khandelwal et al. 2020). Some have recommended 'palliative periodontal treatment' before root hemisection/amputation (Anand et al. 2012b).

Case 24   Hemisection/bicuspidation of the lower molar can result in saving a functional unit. In this case the distal portion of the LR6 was restorable, despite being root canal treated and asymptomatic (Fig. 9.4a, b). Hemisection (Fig. 9.5a, b), endodontic retreatment and a cuspal coverage restoration (Fig. 9.6a) conforming to the occlusion resulted in the patient maintaining a distal contact with the UR5 (Fig. 9.6b).

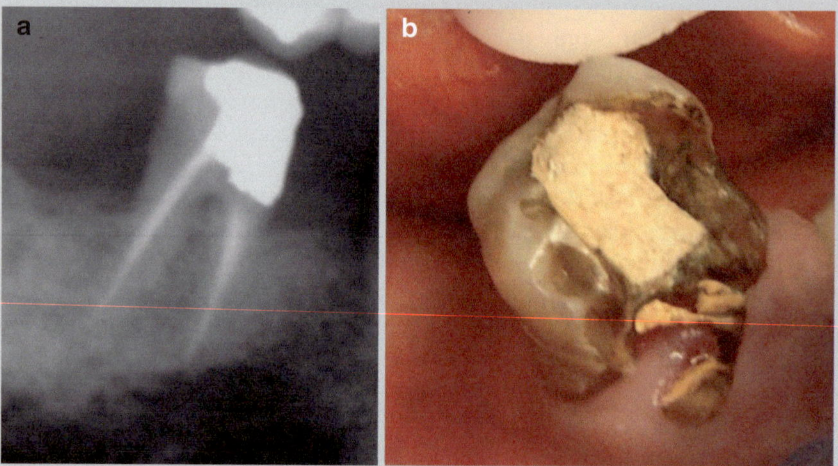

Fig. 9.4   (**a**) LCPA radiograph of the LR6. (**b**) Intra-oral photograph of the LR6 with exposed GP in the mesial canals and a temporary restoration in situ

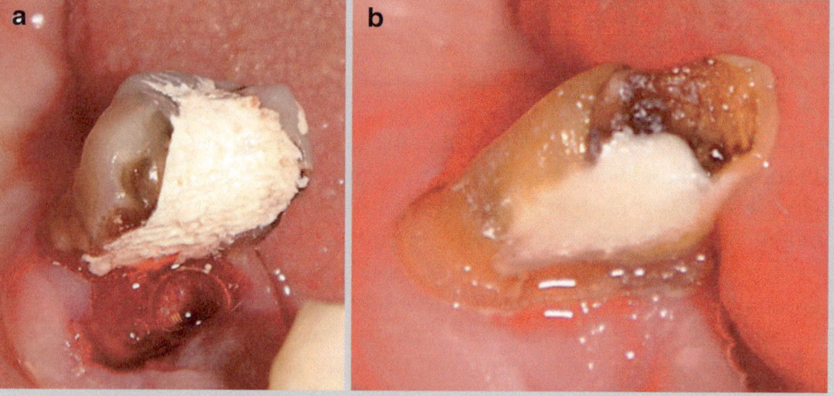

Fig. 9.5   (**a**) Intra-oral photograph of the LR6 having been hemisected and the mesial portion extracted. (**b**) Intra-oral photograph of the now premolar sized LR6 after endodontic treatment and definitive filling placed

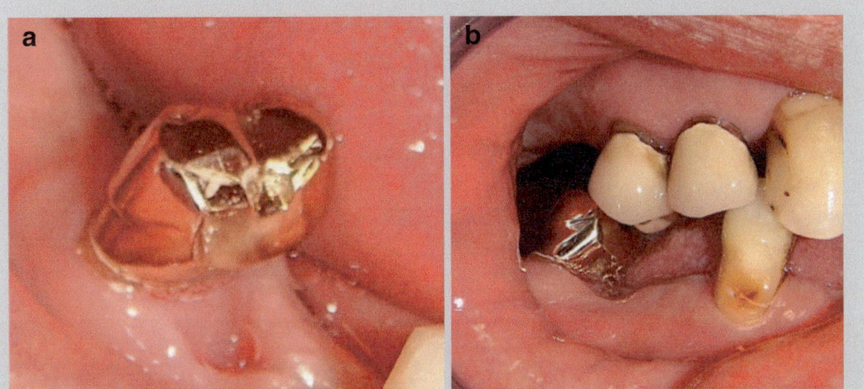

Fig. 9.6 (**a**) Intra-oral photograph of the premolar sized LR6 restored with a milled gold full coverage crown. (**b**) Intra-oral photograph of the LR6 in contact with the UR5 in retruded contact position

The Treatment of Developmental Grooves

When bacteria contaminate developmental grooves, an infrabony defect along the whole length of the groove is possible. The patient is likely to present with a localised periodontal pocket, with or without involvement of the pulp, depending on the extent of the groove and chronicity of the pocket. Radiographically, the groove may be visible as a dark line or as a tear drop shaped radiolucency (Rotstein and Simon 2004). The prognosis is guarded, as it is dependent on the clinician's ability to clean the groove and patient's ability to clean this periodontal pocket and prevent reestablishment of bacteria within the groove. Depending on the extent of a developmental groove, the required treatment may be: (a) non-surgical periodontal treatment if the groove caused a periodontal pocket but does not extend to the pulp chamber or canal system, or (b) non-surgical periodontal treatment and endodontic treatment if the pulp tissue has been reached (Case 25). In some circumstances, it may be appropriate to gain surgical access and possibly to either perform odontoplasty or attempt sealing of the groove (Attam et al. 2010; Santos et al. 2007; Alkan et al. 2006; Schafer et al. 2000; Kim et al. 2017; Alizadeh Tabari et al. 2016). Teeth with palatogingival grooves have also been treated with guided tissue regeneration following root canal treatment, open flap debridement, odontoplasty with or without surgical endodontics (Cho et al. 2017; Miao et al. 2015).

Case 25 The UR2 developed a palatal swelling with repeated drainage (Fig. 9.7). Recession of 2 mm was seen around the tooth with no associated deep periodontal pockets. The UR2 was not tender to percussion, was not responsive to sensibility testing and was of mobility grade I. Generally, good bone levels were seen. Despite root canal treatment, the pocket and apical area remained. Placement of a GP point into the pocket tracked to periradicular and periapical radiolucencies (Fig. 9.8). What are the reasons for this non-healing lesion?

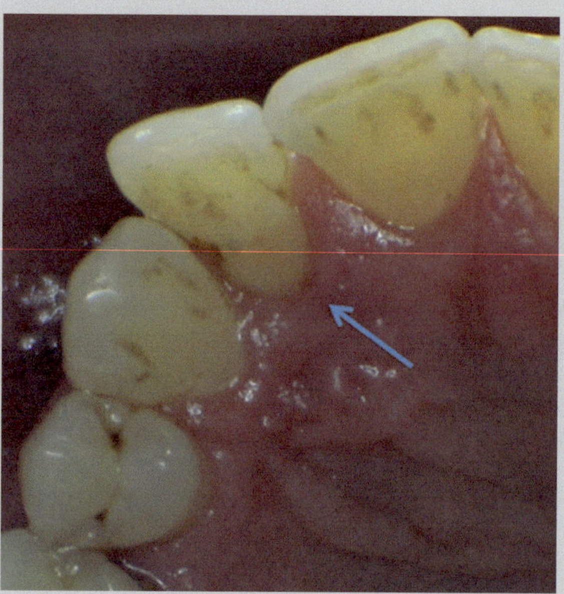

Fig. 9.7 Intra-oral photograph of the UR2 with a palatal groove. The blue arrow points to the periodontal pocket adjacent to a possible crack or groove in the root

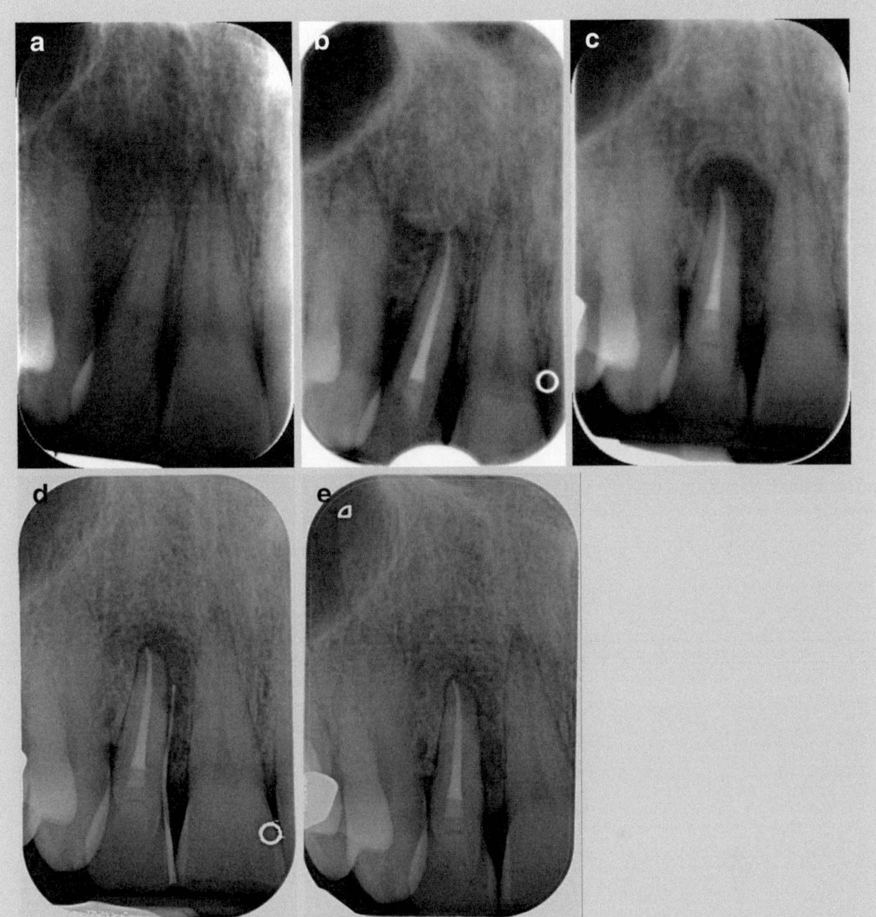

Fig. 9.8 LCPA radiographs of the UR2: (**a**) pre-operatively (Feb 2015), (**b**) following root canal treatment (Jul 2015), (**c**) following root canal re-treatment (Jul 2019), (**d**) at 18 month review (Dec 2020) and (**e**) 30 month review (Dec 2021) following endodontic re-treatment. At review in Dec 2021, there were no deep periodontal pockets and it was not possible to place a GP point into sinus entrance on the mesio palatal aspects of the UR2 (Fig. 9.8e). The tooth had been asymptomatic without suppuration or flare up

Orthodontic Extrusion

Orthodontic extrusion aims to bring the perforation, root fracture, endo-perio lesion supracrestal and bring the gingival architecture with it. However, extrusion in the presence of inflammation can make the osseous defect larger. Often, the tissue appears red and inflamed due to the junctional epithelium, which is non-keratinised with the vasculature visible, after 4 weeks this becomes keratinised, improving the appearance. Even without orthodontic extrusion, on occasion, the periodontal architecture re-establishes below the level of repaired lesions (Fig. 9.9).

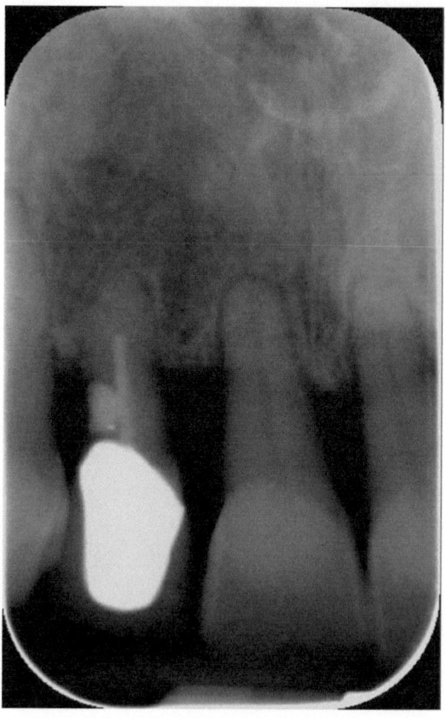

Fig. 9.9 LCPA radiograph of the UR12. Sometimes following periodontal treatment, healing of the soft tissues leads to resorption defects or perforation becoming more coronal

The Use of Antibiotics in the Management of Perio-Endo Lesions

Local and systemic antimicrobial adjuncts to debridement may be advantageous for periodontal treatment (Herrera et al. 2020), however in perio-endo lesions, removing the source of infection through mechanical/chemo-mechanical means is preferred. Systemic antibiotics should only be considered in cases where spreading infection is likely, especially where surgical incision and draining is not possible (Anand et al. 2012b).

Splinting and the Management of Perio-Endo Lesions

Mobility of teeth can be as a result of a number of factors including root or crown fracture, apical pathology, overloading of teeth with good bone support (primary occlusal trauma) or as a result of periodontal breakdown and reduced bone support unable to cope with the normal occlusal loads (secondary occlusal trauma). Mobility of teeth as a result of resorption is rare. Some have thought that excessive occlusal forces can exacerbate periodontal breakdown through an altered pathway of periodontal destruction and have demonstrated this in animals (Glickman et al. 1961; Glickman and Smulow 1965) and others have disputed this, suggesting that inflammation and bone loss was associated with the presence of plaque (Waerhaug 1979). Studies have shown that occlusal adjustment, where necessary, as part of surgical and non-surgical periodontal treatment gave better healing outcomes (Burgett et al. 1992; McGuire and Nunn 1996a, b; Sonnenschein et al. 2021). Mobility alone however, has been shown not to lead to tooth loss, and mobile teeth can be maintained long-term, even without splinting (Hirschfeld and Wasserman 1978; Polson 1980).

The reason for mobility must be assessed and potential causes must be treated: such as root canal treatment for teeth with apical pathology, occlusal adjustment for teeth exhibiting fremitus and periodontal treatment with improvement in oral hygiene to remove plaque. Where tooth mobility remains, splinting teeth may be an option. Splinting of mobile periodontally involved teeth has been practiced for many years (Tarnow and Fletcher 1986). If mobility of a tooth is related to occlusal trauma and occlusal adjustment is possible to eliminate fremitus, this is preferred as a splint may lead to additional difficulties with maintain good oral hygiene. However, if the tooth mobility is related to the level of bone loss, such that the normal forces during function exacerbate the movement, splinting to adjacent teeth may be of advantage, for example, Case 26 (Kathariya et al. 2016). High survival rates for such teeth (80%) at 5 years have been reported (Quirynen et al. 1999).

Case 26 A periodontally susceptible female patient, aged 35 years, presented with a 10 mm periodontal pocket and 3 mm of recession associated with the LL1, which displayed grade 1 mobility (Fig. 9.10a). The LL1 gave a positive response to sensibility testing and was not tender to percussion. Following non-surgical periodontal treatment and splinting to the adjacent teeth (carried out by her general dental practitioner), the periodontal pocket resolved to 4 mm with 3 mm of recession. The LL1 continues to respond positively to sensibility testing without associated symptoms. The LL1 may have appeared to be periodontally and endodontically involved, however as can be seen with careful examination of the pre-operative radiograph, the apical area may not yet be involved. With the tooth testing positively with sensibility testing, splinting of the LL1 was a wise choice, and shows the potential for bony infill with good plaque control, periodontal treatment and reducing the movement of the tooth while healing (Fig. 9.10b).

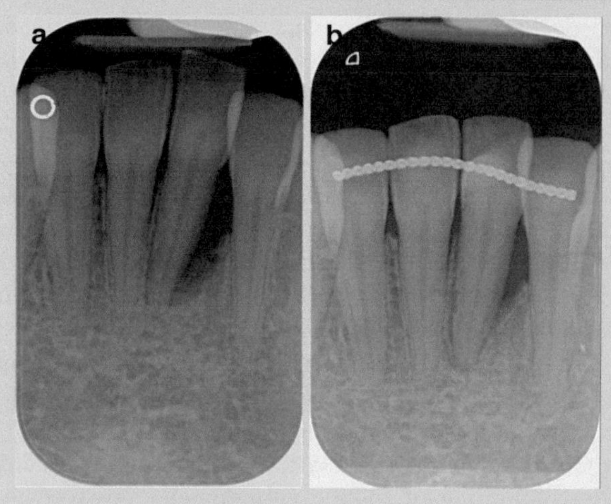

Fig. 9.10 LCPA radiographs of the LL1 (**a**) pre-operatively (Jan 2021), (**b**) following splinting of the lower central and lateral incisors (Dec 2021)

Contra-Indications for Dental Extractions

There are a growing number of patients who are surviving longer, following radiotherapy for head and neck cancer and there are a growing number of patients who are taking anti-angiogenic medication such as bisphosphonates. Although the pathophysiology may be different, the outcome for both these groups of patients is the delay and possible non-healing of the alveolar bone, should dental extractions or surgical treatment be performed. The exposed bone is susceptible to infections that can be painful and affect the patient's quality of life (Eliyas and Porter 2020).

These patients may present with pain that mimics endodontic disease, or with suppuration that mimics periodontal disease. Often the teeth test positively to sensibility testing, although the patient may present with dull aching pain, affecting a number of teeth in any quadrant and numerous teeth may be tender to percussion. Instigation of root canal treatment will not resolve the symptoms, however this treatment is required if there is any doubt regarding endodontic infection. The osteonecrosis may eventually present as a perio-endo lesion.

Case 27 This 62-year old male presented, prior to starting intravenous bisphosphonates for myeloma (Fig. 9.11a). He agreed to have the LL7 removed before oncology treatment, as the restorability was unknown, but chose to keep the LL6. More than 14 days of healing were allowed prior to starting intravenous bisphosphonates. He also underwent periodontal treatment and oral health education. He then presented almost 2 years later, with a

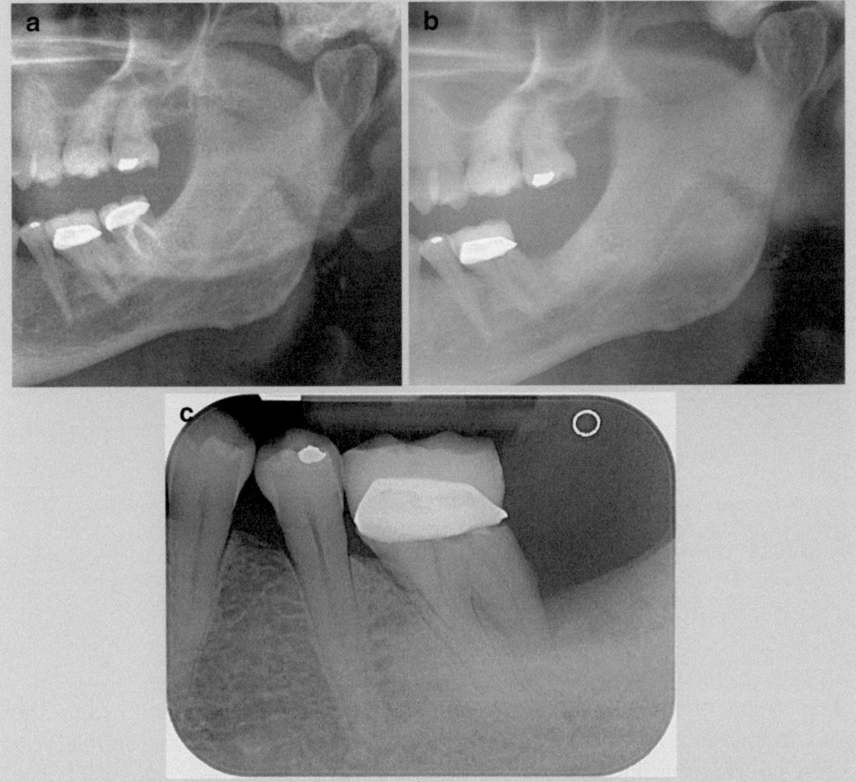

Fig. 9.11 (a) Sectional DPT of the left side taken in Aug 2017 showing heavily restored LL67. (b) Sectional DPT of the left side taken in May 2019 showed no obvious pathology in the lower left quadrant. (c) LCPA radiograph of the LL6 (Oct 2020) showing 60% horizontal bone loss on the distal aspect without obvious apical pathology

dull aching pain from the lower left quadrant (Fig. 9.11b). The patient was sure that the cause of the pain was the LL6, although, this tooth was not tender to percussion. Sensibility testing results were mixed from the LL6, 50% bone loss and furcation involvement (grade 1) were seen, without associated deep pockets (Fig. 9.11c). As 20% of crowned teeth could lose vitality, it is possible that part of the pulpal tissue may have lost vitality. What are the possible diagnoses for the LL6? (Fig. 9.12)

The patient was very keen to remove the crown and investigate the LL6, although, the symptoms may not have been associated with the LL6. Luckily the tooth was restorable, and endodontic treatment was instigated (Fig. 9.12). The tooth was vital on entry. The area remained symptomatic and despite several appointments to clean and dress the tooth. As time progressed, it became more evident that the symptoms were related to bisphosphonate related osteonecrosis of the jaws (BRONJ). Despite the lack of improvement in symptoms, root canal and periodontal treatment were completed. The symptoms were temporarily treated with antibiotics, however, is more than likely to recur. This case highlights how difficult it can be to decipher between endodontic symptoms, and that related to anti-angiogenic medication.

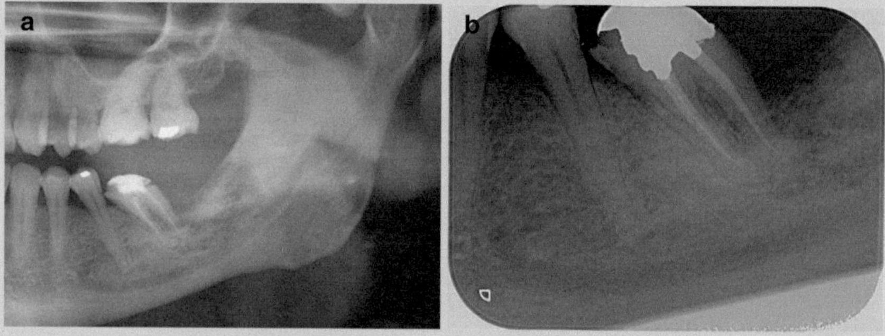

Fig. 9.12 (**a**) Sectional DPT of the left side taken in Apr 2021 showing significant bony changes despite the LL6 having been root canal treated. (**b**) LCPA radiograph of the LL6 (Apr 2021) showing 60% bone loss on the distal aspect of the LL6 and bony changes that can be mistaken for periapical pathology

The affects of radiotherapy on pulps have been inconclusive, with some showing no change in pulp, others showing decreased pulpal sensitivity and decreased oxygen saturation after radiotherapy (Knowles et al. 1986; Kataoka et al. 2011). When endodontic treatment is required for patients post radiotherapy to the jaws, the use of local anaesthetic without vasoconstrictors is recommended, especially in the mandible, and this may be beneficial for periodontal treatment also. Care must be taken not to traumatise the gingival tissues during treatment (such as the use of rubber dam clamps subgingivally) as this may lead to osteoradionecrosis (ORN). Equally care should be taken during provision of non-surgical periodontal therapy for the same reason. In such patients, treatments like crown lengthening surgery and periodontal surgery may carry high risks of non-healing, and therefore, should be considered very carefully (Irie et al. 2018). Similar precautions may be required for patients on anti-angiogenic medication also. In these patients, extractions are contraindicated wherever possible, and therefore, the provision of non-surgical periodontal and endodontic treatment will be the only option. It should be accepted that by definition, the healing ability of the bone in these patients is impaired, and as such, it may appear that lesions are not healing (Fig. 9.13). Provision of dental treatment may prevent or delay infection of the bone that may lead to the development of ORN or medication related osteonecrosis of the jaws (MRONJ).

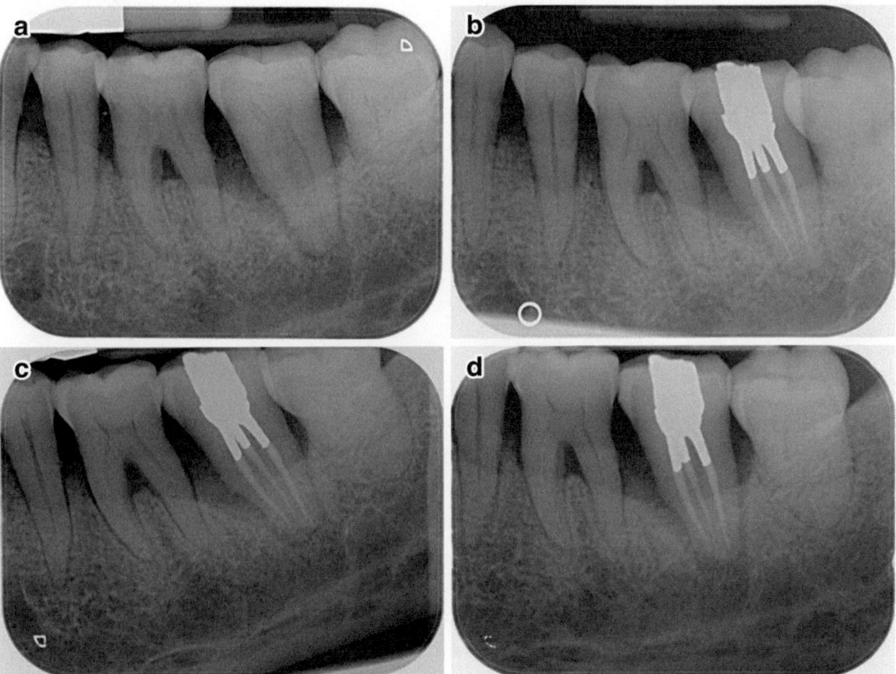

Fig. 9.13 LCPA radiographs of the LL7: A 62-year-old female patient presented with 4-5mm pockets on mesial, distal and lingual aspects of the LL7 (**a**). Following urgent root canal treatment and root surface debridement in preparation for a stem cell transplant (**b**), the pocket reduced to a single 5mm pocket on the mesiolingual aspect of the LL7. Despite 3monthly periodontal treatment the patient has struggled to improve the periodontal pockets, which has oscillated between 3-5mm depending on the oral hygiene. The LL7 has remained grade I mobile but not tender to percussion, without change in the apical area at 1 year review (**c**), but with development of an apical radiolucency at the two-year review (**d**). The patient has been having monthly intravenous bisphosphonates for many years, and this non-healing may be related to MRONJ

Case 28 A head and neck cancer patient who has undergone radiotherapy to the jaws: This patient had a susceptibility to periodontal disease and this progressed during radiotherapy. Extraction is not an option, therefore, endodontic treatment and regular periodontal debridement is all that can be offered. There is a risk of ORN with extraction, although, periodontal and endodontic treatment may not lead to healing due the compromised blood supply to the mandible after radiotherapy (Fig. 9.14). This could already be ORN, and LR7 may also require periodontal and endodontic treatment in due course. Should these teeth have been extracted prior to radiotherapy?

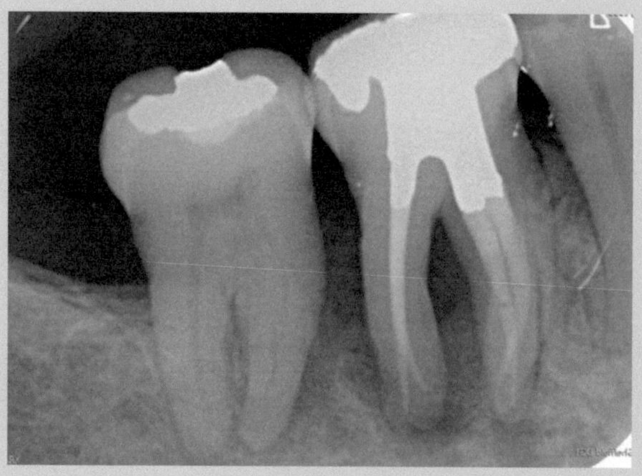

Fig. 9.14 LCPA radiograph of the LR67. The LR6 has been root canal treated. There is horizontal and vertical bone loss associate with both the LR6 and LR7

Case 29 This 47-year old patient presented with aching pain in the upper right quadrant (Fig. 9.15a). The medical history included breast cancer and treatment with intravenous Zolendronic acid to manage metastases to the bone. A diagnosis of apical periodontitis as a result of a failed root canal treatment in the UR6 was made. The UR6 was carious and initially restored to facilitate a seal during root canal re-treatment. Root canal treatment of the UR6 was then delayed due to medical treatment. When the patient then presented a few months later (Fig. 9.15b), the UR5 was almost devoid of bone as seen radiographically, with exposed bone around the full circumference of the root, clinically. Several months later the UR5 and the exposed bone exfoliated, leaving a well-healed ridge and relieving the patient of pain. Endodontic treatment of the UR6 and periodontal treatment was completed, and the patient continues to be asymptomatic, without further exposed bone (Fig. 9.16).

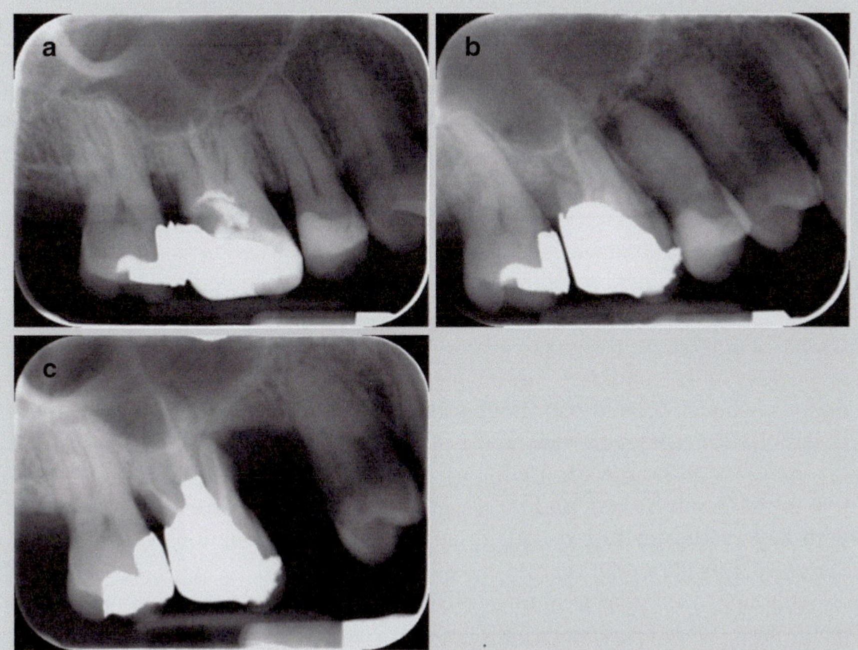

Fig. 9.15 LCPA radiograph of the UR4567: (**a**) showing a scantily condensed root filling in the UR6 without any obvious pathology associated with the UR45 (January 2018). (**b**) Showing significant bone loss associated with the UR5 within 6 months (June 2018) and (**c**) following exfoliation of the UR5 and completion of the endodontic re-treatment of the UR6 (September 2019)

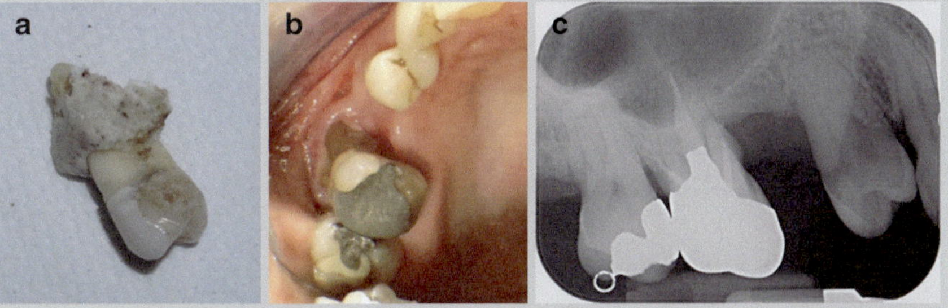

Fig. 9.16 (**a**) Photograph of the exfoliated UR5 and bone. (**b**) Intra-oral photograph of the healed UR5 site. (**c**) LCPA radiograph of the UR4567 showing no further deterioration (January 2021)

The presence of unmanaged periodontal and endodontic treatment pre-radiotherapy leads to delayed healing (Schuurhuis et al. 2018). The presence of periodontal and endodontic infection in those taking anti-angiogenic medication has the potential to lead to MRONJ. It is difficult to know the likelihood of healing following root canal treatment and periodontal treatment in those who have undergone radiotherapy to the jaws or those who have taken anti-angiogenic medication.

Case 30 This 46-year old male patient presented for dental assessment prior to starting intravenous bisphosphonates for multiple myeloma. The only restoration present was a small buccal cervical composite restoration on the UL4. There were mild signs of attrition, erosion and abrasion, with periodontal pockets of 4–5 mm. None of the teeth were mobile or tender to percussion, there was no associated soft tissue swellings, sinus or tenderness. Multi-foci of radiolucent areas were seen in the mandible as a result of myeloma, resorbing the roots of the LR456, LL7 (Fig. 9.17a, b). None of the teeth were positive to the Tooth Slooth, and no obvious fracture lines were seen associated with any of the teeth. No soft tissues sings of parafunction were present, therefore, this parafunction may have been historical.

Although it may be tempting to consider endodontic treatment for these teeth, these bony lesions are not dental infections, and accessing these teeth for endodontic treatment may increase the chance of introducing pathogens to an otherwise sterile area. It is imperative that the periodontal disease is stabilised with non-surgical treatment and improvement in oral hygiene, as to avoid progression to perio-endo lesions. This patient was urgently given intravenous bisphosphonates to manage the myeloma, and will be carefully monitored from a dental perspective. Change in the bony lesions following myeloma treatment is evident when comparing the pre-myeloma treatment and post-myeloma treatment radiographs (Fig. 9.18a, b).

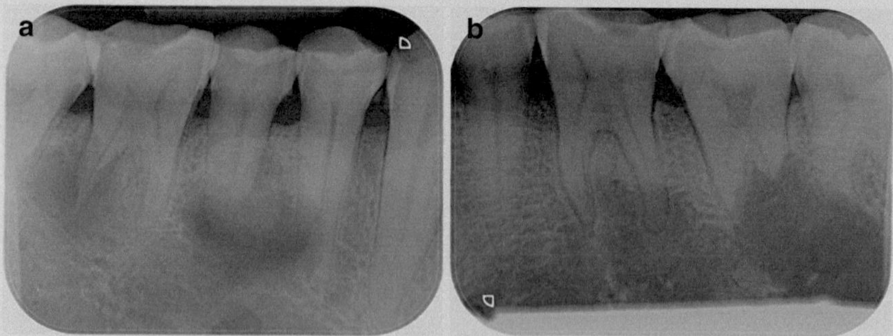

Fig. 9.17 LCPA radiographs of (**a**) the LR456 and (**b**) the LL567, showing radiolucencies and root resorption of the unrestored LR654, LL7

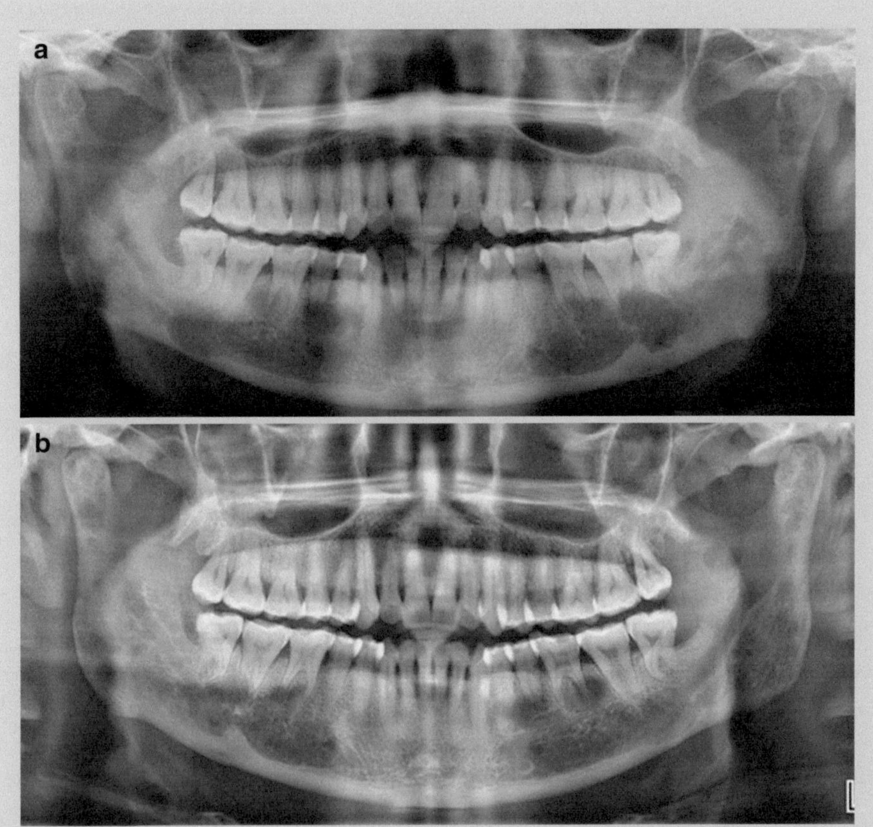

Fig. 9.18 DPTs showing (**a**) the presence of generalised root resorption and apical radiolucencies pre-myeloma treatment (2021) and (**b**) the resolution of some of the radiolucencies post-myeloma treatment (2022)

References

Abbott P. Endodontic management of combined endodontic- periodontal lesions. J N Z Soc Periodontol. 1998;83:15–28.

Abbott PV, Salgado JC. Strategies for the endodontic management of concurrent endodontic and periodontal diseases. Aust Dent J. 2009;54:S70–85.

Alizadeh Tabari Z, Homayouni H, Pourseyediyan T, Arvin A, Eiland D, Moradi MN. Treatment of a developmental groove and supernumerary root using guided tissue regeneration technique. Case Rep Dent. 2016;2016:2738569.

Alkan A, Keskiner I, Yuzbasioglu E. Connective tissue grafting on resin ionomer in localized gingival recession. J Periodontol. 2006;77:1446–51.

Anand V, Govila V, Gulati M. Endo-perio lesion: part i (the pathogenesis) – a review. Arch Dent Sci. 2012a;3(1):3–9.

Anand V, Govila V, Gulati M. Endo-perio lesion: part ii (the treatment) – a review. Arch Dent Sci. 2012b;3(1):10–6.

Attam K, Tiwary R, Talwar S, Lamba AK. Palatogingival groove: endodontic-periodontal management – case report. J Endod. 2010;36:1717–20.

Bergenholtz A. Radectomy of multirooted teeth. J Am Dent Assoc. 1972;85(4):870–5.

Blomlöf L, Lindskog S, Hammarstrom L. Influence of pulpal treatments on cell and tissue reactions in the marginal periodontium. J Periodontol. 1988;59:577–83.

Blomlöf L, Jansson L, Appelgren R, Ehnevid H, Lindskog S. Prognosis and mortality of root-resected molars. Int J Periodontics Restorative Dent. 1997;17(2):190–201.

Bühler H. Evaluation of root-resected teeth. Results after 10 years. J Periodontol. 1988;59(12):805–10.

Burgett FG, Ramfjord SP, Nissle RR, Morrison EC, Charbeneau TD, Caffesse RG. A randomized trial of occlusal adjustment in the treatment of periodontitis patients. J Clin Periodontol. 1992;19(6):381–7.

Carnevale G, Di Febo G, Tonelli MP, Marin C, Fuzzi M. A retrospective analysis of the periodontal-prosthetic treatment of molars with interradicular lesions. Int J Periodontics Restorative Dent. 1991;11(3):189–205.

Carnevale G, Pontoriero R, di Febo G. Long-term effects of root-resective therapy in furcation-involved molars. A 10-year longitudinal study. J Clin Periodontol. 1998;25(3):209–14.

Chapple ILC, Lumley PJ. The perio-endo interface. Dent Update. 1999;26:331–41.

Cho YD, Lee JE, Chung Y, Lee WC, Seol YJ, Lee YM, Rhyu IC, Ku Y. Collaborative management of combined periodontal-endodontic lesions with a palatogingival groove: a case series. J Endod. 2017;43(2):332–7.

Cortellini P, Stalpers G, Mollo A, Tonetti MS. Periodontal regeneration versus extraction and prosthetic replacement of teeth severely compromised by attachment loss to the apex: 5-year results of an ongoing randomized clinical trial. J Clin Periodontol. 2011;38(10):915–24.

Cortellini P, Stalpers G, Mollo A, Tonetti MS. Periodontal regeneration versus extraction and dental implant or prosthetic replacement of teeth severely compromised by attachment loss to the apex: a randomized controlled clinical trial reporting 10-year outcomes, survival analysis and mean cumulative cost of recurrence. J Clin Periodontol. 2020;47(6):768–76.

Dongari A, Lambrianidis T. Periodontally derived pulpal lesions. Endod Dent Traumatol. 1988;4:49–54.

Ehnevid H, Jansson L, Lindskog S, Blomlof L. Periodontal healing in teeth with periapical lesions. A clinical retrospective study. J Clin Periodontol. 1993;20:254–8.

Eliyas S, Porter R. An impossible choice: MRONJ vs. ORN? The difficulties of the decision-making process for head and neck cancer patients on long-term anti-angiogenic medication. Br Dent J. 2020;229(9):587–90.

Fang F, Gao B, He T, Lin Y. Efficacy of root canal therapy combined with basic periodontal therapy and its impact on inflammatory responses in patients with combined periodontal-endodontic lesions. Am J Transl Res. 2021;13(12):14149–56.

Filipowicz F, Umstott P, England M. Vital root resection in maxillary molar teeth: a longitudinal study. J Endod. 1984;10:264–8.

Friedrich F, Scalabrin SA, Weissheimer T, Rösing CK, Só GB, da Rosa RA, Só MVR. Influence of the timing of periodontal intervention on periapical/periodontal repair in endodontic-periodontal lesions: a systematic review. Clin Oral Investig. 2023;27(3):933–42.

Fugazzotto PA. A comparison of the success of root resected molars and molar position implants in function in a private practice: results of up to 15-plus years. J Periodontol. 2001;72(8):1113–23.

Glickman I, Smulow JB. Effect of excessive occlusal forces upon the pathway of gingival inflammation in humans. J Periodontol. 1965;36:141–7.

Glickman I, Stein S, Smulow J. The effect of increased functional forces upon the periodontium of splinted and non-splinted teeth. J Periodontol. 1961;32:290–300.

Gupta S, Tewari S, Mittal S. Effect of the time lapse between endodontic and periodontal therapies on the healing of concurrent endodontic-periodontal lesions without communication: a prospective randomized clinical trial. J Endod. 2015;41:785–90.

Herrera D, Matesanz P, Martín C, Oud V, Feres M, Teughels W. Adjunctive effect of locally delivered antimicrobials in periodontitis therapy: a systematic review and meta-analysis. J Clin Periodontol. 2020;47(Suppl 22):239–56.

Hirschfeld L, Wasserman B. A long-term survey of tooth loss in 600 treated periodontal patients. J Periodontol. 1978;49:225–37.

Irie MS, Mendes EM, Borges JS, Osuna LG, Rabelo GD, Soares PB. Periodontal therapy for patients before and after radiotherapy: a review of the literature and topics of interest for clinicians. Med Oral Pathol Oral Cir Bucal. 2018;23(5):e524–30.

Jansson L, Ehnevid H, Lindskog S, Blomlof L. Relationship between periapical and periodontal status. A clinical retrospective study. J Clin Periodontol. 1993;20:117–23.

Jansson L, Ehnevid H, Blomlof L, Weintraub A, et al. Endodontic pathogens in periodontal disease augmentation. J Clin Periodontol. 1995;22:598–602.

Jaoui L, Machtou P, Ouhayoun JP. Long-term evaluation of endodontic and periodontal treatment. Int Endod J. 1995;28:249–54.

Kataoka SH, Setzer FC, Gondim-Junior E, Pessoa OF, Gavini G, Caldeira CL. Pulp vitality in patients with intraoral and oropharyngeal malignant tumors undergoing radiation therapy assessed by pulse oximetry. J Endod. 2011;37(9):1197–200.

Kathariya R, Devanoorkar A, Golani R, Shetty N, Vallakatla V, Bhat MY. To splint or not to splint: the current status of periodontal splinting. J Int Acad Periodontol. 2016;18(2):45–56.

Kerekes K, Olsen I. Similarities in the microflora of root canals and deep periodontal pockets. Endod Dent Traumatol. 1990;6:1–5.

Khandelwal A, Billore J, Gupta B, Jaroli S, Agrawal N. Knowledge, attitude and perception on endo-perio lesions in practicing dentists – a qualitative research study. J Adv Med Dent Sci Res. 2020;11(8):31–4.

Kim E, Song JS, Jung IY, Lee SJ, Kim S. Prospective clinical study evaluating endodontic microsurgery outcomes for cases with lesions of endodontic origin compared with cases with lesions of combined periodontal-endodontic origin. J Endod. 2008;34(5):546–51.

Kim HJ, Choi Y, Yu MK, Lee KW, Min KS. Recognition and management of palatogingival groove for tooth survival: a literature review. Restor Dent Endod. 2017;42(2):77–86.

Kinsel RP, Lamb RE, Ho D. The treatment dilemma of the furcated molar: root resection versus single-tooth implant restoration. A literature review. Int J Oral Maxillofac Implants. 1998;13(3):322–32. Erratum in: Int J Oral Maxillofac Implants 1998;13(5):720

Kipioti A, Nakou M, Legakis N, Mitsis F. Microbiological findings of infected root canals and adjacent periodontal pockets in teeth with advanced periodontitis. Oral Surg Oral Med Oral Pathol. 1984;58:213–20.

Knowles JC, Chalian VA, Shidnia H. Pulp innervation after radiation therapy. J Prosthet Dent. 1986;56(6):708–11.

Kobayashi T, Hayashi A, Yoshikawa R, Okuda K, Hara K. The microbial flora from root canals and periodontal pockets of non-vital teeth associated with advanced periodontitis. Int Endod J. 1990;23(2):100–6.

Kurihara H, Kobayashi Y, Francisco LA, Isoshima O, Nagai A, Murayama Y. A microbiological and immunological study of endodontic-periodontic lesions. J Endod. 1995;21:617–21.

Langer B, Stein SD, Wagenberg B. An evaluation of root resections. A ten-year study. J Periodontol. 1981;52(12):719–22.

Lindskog S, Lengheden A, Blomlöf L. Successive removal of periodontal tissues. Marginal healing without plaque control. J Clin Periodontol. 1993;20:14–9.

McGuire MK, Nunn ME. Prognosis versus actual outcome. II. The effectiveness of clinical parameters in developing an accurate prognosis. J Periodontol. 1996a;67(7):658–65.

McGuire MK, Nunn ME. Prognosis versus actual outcome. III. The effectiveness of clinical parameters in accurately predicting tooth survival. J Periodontol. 1996b;67(7):666–74.

Miao H, Chen M, Otgonbayar T, Zhang SS, Hou MH, Wu Z, Wang YL, Wu LG. Papillary reconstruction and guided tissue regeneration for combined periodontal-endodontic lesions caused by palatogingival groove and additional root: a case report. Clin Case Rep. 2015;3(12): 1042–9.

Miyashita H, Bergenholtz G, Grondohl K, Wennestrom JL. Impact of endodontic conditions on marginal bone loss. J Periodontol. 1998;69:158–64.

Odell EW, Cawson RA. In: Odell EW, editor. Cawson's essentials of oral pathology and oral medicine. 9th ed. Amsterdam: Elsevier; 2017.

Park SY, Shin SY, Yang SM, Kye SB. Factors influencing the outcome of root-resection therapy in molars: a 10-year retrospective study. J Periodontol. 2009;80(1):32–40.

Polson AM. Interrelationship of inflammation and tooth mobility (trauma) in pathogenesis of periodontal disease. J Clin Periodontol. 1980;7(5):351–60.

Quirynen M, Mongardini C, Lambrechts P, et al. A long-term evaluation of composite bonded natural/resin teeth as replacement of lower incisors with terminal periodontitis. J Periodontol. 1999;702:205–12.

Rosen E, Tsesis I, Kavalerchik E, Salem R, Kahn A, Del Fabbro M, Taschieri S, Corbella S. Effect of guided tissue regeneration on the success of surgical endodontic treatment of teeth with endodontic-periodontal lesions: A systematic review. Int Endod J. 2023;56(8):910–21.

Rotstein I, Simon JH. Diagnosis, prognosis and decision- making in the treatment of combined periodontal-endodontic lesions. Periodontol. 2004;34:165–203.

Santos VR, Lucchesi JA, Cortelli SC, Amaral CM, Feres M, Duarte PM. Effects of glass ionomer and microfilled composite subgingival restorations on periodontal tissue and subgingival biofilm: a 6-month evaluation. J Periodontol. 2007;78:1522–8.

Schacher B, Haueisen H, Ratka-Krueger P. The chicken or the egg? Periodontal-endodontic lesions. PERIO. 2007;4:15–21.

Schafer E, Cankay R, Ott K. Malformations in maxillary incisors: case report of radicular palatal groove. Dent Traumatol. 2000;16(3):132–7.

Schmidt JC, Walter C, Amato M, Weiger R. Treatment of periodontal-endodontic lesions--a systematic review. J Clin Periodontol. 2014;41(8):779–90.

Schuurhuis JM, Stokman MA, Witjes MJH, Reintsema H, Langendijk JA, Vissink A, Spijkervet FKL. Patients with advanced periodontal disease before intensity-modulated radiation therapy are prone to develop bone-healing problems: a 2-year prospective follow-up study. Support Care Cancer. 2018;26(4):1133–42.

Song M, Kang M, Kang DR, Jung HI, Kim E. Comparison of the effect of endodontic-periodontal combined lesion on the outcome of endodontic microsurgery with that of isolated endodontic lesion: survival analysis using propensity score analysis. Clin Oral Investig. 2018;22(4):1717–24.

Sonnenschein SK, Ciardo A, Kilian S, Ziegler P, Ruetters M, Splindler M, Kim TS. The impact of splinting time point of mobile mandibular incisors on the outcome of periodontal treatment-preliminary observations from a randomized clinical trial. Clin Oral Investig. 2021;26:1–10.

Sundqvist G. Associations between microbial species in dental root canal infections. Oral Microbiol Immunol. 1992;7:257–62.

Tarnow DP, Fletcher P. Splinting of periodontally involved teeth: indications and contraindications. N Y State Dent J. 1986;52(5):24–5.

Trope M, Yesilsoy C, Koren L, Moshonov J, Friedman S. Effect of different endodontic treatment protocols on periodontal repair and root resorption of replanted dog teeth. J Endod. 1992;18(10):492–6.

Ustaoğlu G, Uğur Aydin Z, Özelçi F. Comparison of GTR, T-PRF and open-flap debridement in the treatment of intrabony defects with endo-perio lesions: a randomized controlled trial. Med Oral Patol Oral Cir Bucal. 2020;25(1):e117–23.

Vakalis SV, Whitworth JM, Ellwood RP, Preshaw PM. A pilot study of treatment of periodontal-endodontic lesions. Int Dent J. 2005;55(5):313–8.

Waerhaug J. The infrabony pocket and its relationship to trauma from occlusion and subgingival plaque. J Periodontol. 1979;507:355–65.

Whyman RA. Endodontic-periodontic lesions. Part 2; management. N Z Dent J. 1988;85:109–11.

Zehnder M, Gold SI, Hasselgren G. Pathologic interaction in pulpal and periodontal tissues. J Clin Periodontol. 2002;29:663–71.

Summary for Diagnosing and Treating Perio-Endo Lesions

10

Abstract

The diagnosis of perio-endo lesions is important for formulating a plan of treatment and making a decision on the prognosis of the tooth. This last chapter summarises the key points to be remembered. The end of this book lists a few questions to test your learning.

Summary of Periodontal Lesions, Endodontic Lesions and Perio-Endo Lesions

At this stage, it is worthwhile remembering the usual symptoms of periodontal lesions, endodontic lesions and compare them to those of perio-endo lesions (Table 10.1).

S. Eliyas, *The Periodontic-Endodontic Interface*,
https://doi.org/10.1007/978-3-031-49937-1_10

Table 10.1 Summary for diagnosis of perio-endo lesions

	Periodontal Lesions	Endodontic Lesions	Perio-Endo Lesions
What are the symptoms?	Usually asymptomatic, patients may report bleeding on probing	Tenderness to bite on. Maybe asymptomatic if chronic and draining sinus present.	May not be tender to bite on, pain may only be present if acute exacerbation, and maybe absent of draining sinus
Will the tooth be tender to percussion?	No, unless there is an acute periodontal abscess, or an acute apical abscess. Patient may report the tooth feeling 'different' when percussed	No, unless there is an acute apical abscess. Patient may report the tooth feeling 'different' when percussed	No, unless there is an acute periodontitis, acute apical abscess or acute periodontal abscess. Patient may report the tooth feeling 'different' when percussed
Other clinical signs	Possible mobility	Possible mobility	Possible mobility
Is the lesion limited to one tooth?	No (unless there is localised periodontal disease, or local factors such as overhangs leading to periodontal breakdown)	Yes	Yes (unless the patient has numerous teeth with, untreated periodontal disease, leading to pulp necrosis and numerous perio-endo lesions)
Does the tooth have extensive caries, restoration, and signs of cracks, root fractures?	No	Yes	Possibly, if the endodontic disease occurred separately to the periodontal disease, was left untreated, and the two lesions combined
Does the tooth respond to sensibility testing?	Yes	No	No
Is there a periodontal probing defect?	Yes, usually a wide based pocket	Possibly, a narrow pocket, if draining through the pocket or near the gingival crevice	Yes, usually a wide based pocket due to the periodontal disease
Is crestal bone loss seen on the radiograph?	Yes	No	Yes, usually a wide vertical defect as well as generalised horizontal bone loss
Is there an apical area present?	No (unless there is superimposition of a deep pocket on the radiographic apex of the tooth)	Yes, usually (however the lesions needs time to show radiographically, and if the cortical bone is thick it may not be seen radiographically)	Yes, often
What are the clinical signs?	Deep periodontal pockets, mobility, sometimes suppuration from pockets	Tenderness to percussion, mobility, possible narrow deep pocket often with suppuration	Deep periodontal pockets, mobility, suppuration, teeth may not necessarily be tender to percussion
What are the microbes present?	More spirochetes, subgingival plaque may house more anaerobic species	Very few species, mostly anaerobic	More microbes and species than in endodontic lesions alone, therefore the microbial load is more complex than in endodontic lesions.

Periodontal Lesions and Primary Periodontal Lesions with a Secondary Endodontic Component

Main Learning Points (Fig. 10.1)

- Periodontal lesions without an endodontic component may show marginal bone loss, as seen radiographically, without extension to the apex. Where as, when there is a secondary endodontic component, there will be marginal bone loss, either localised or generalised, extending to the apex of the root. Both can cause mobility of the tooth.
- If there is an endodontic involvement, the tooth may give a negative response to sensibility testing, however, there may still not be tenderness to percussion as there may be drainage through the periodontal pocket.
- Periodontal lesions will heal with periodontal treatment in motivated patients, however, those with a secondary endodontic component will not heal unless endodontic treatment is also provided.

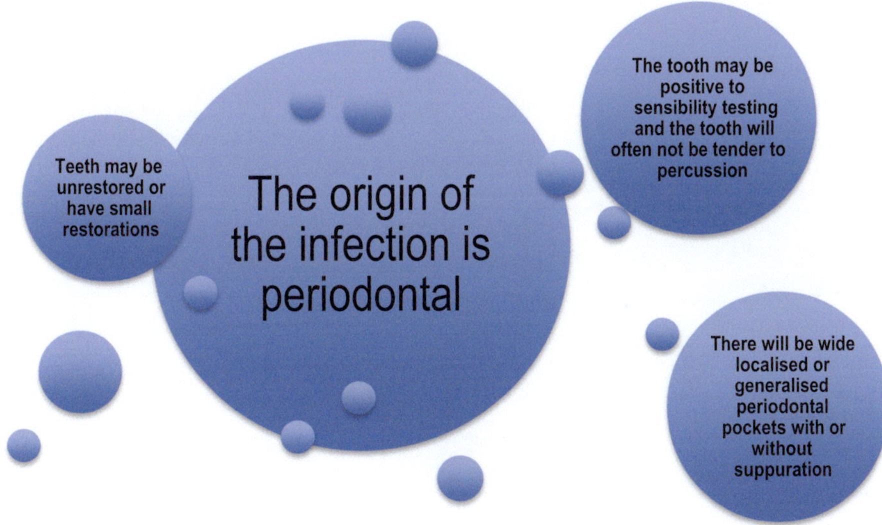

Fig. 10.1 Summary of the main learning points for teeth with a perio-endo lesion

Endodontic Lesions and Primary Endodontic Lesions with a Secondary Periodontal Component

Main Learning Points (Fig. 10.2)

- Reasons for a tooth to lose vitality may be caries, failed restorations, presence of large/deep restorations or crowns, a history of trauma, signs of parafunction that may indicate the presence of a crack.
- Endodontic lesions without a periodontal component may show a draining sinus close to the gingival crevice or a narrow periodontal pocket, without significant marginal bone loss as seen radiographically. Where there is a secondary periodontal component, there may be marginal bone loss, either localised or generalised. Both can cause mobility of the tooth.
- Endodontic lesions will heal with endodontic treatment, however, if there is an established secondary periodontal component, periodontal treatment will also be required.

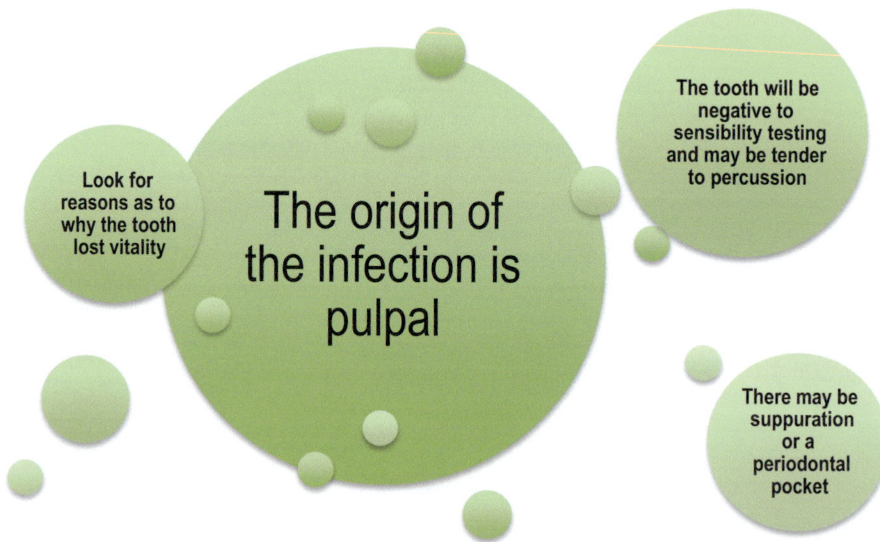

Fig. 10.2 Summary of the main learning points for teeth with an endo-perio lesion

Concomitant and Combined Lesions

Concomitant and combined lesions can look very much the same clinically, and the only deciding factor may be the radiographic appearance, although often with established lesions, it may not be possible to differentiate the two (Fig. 10.3).

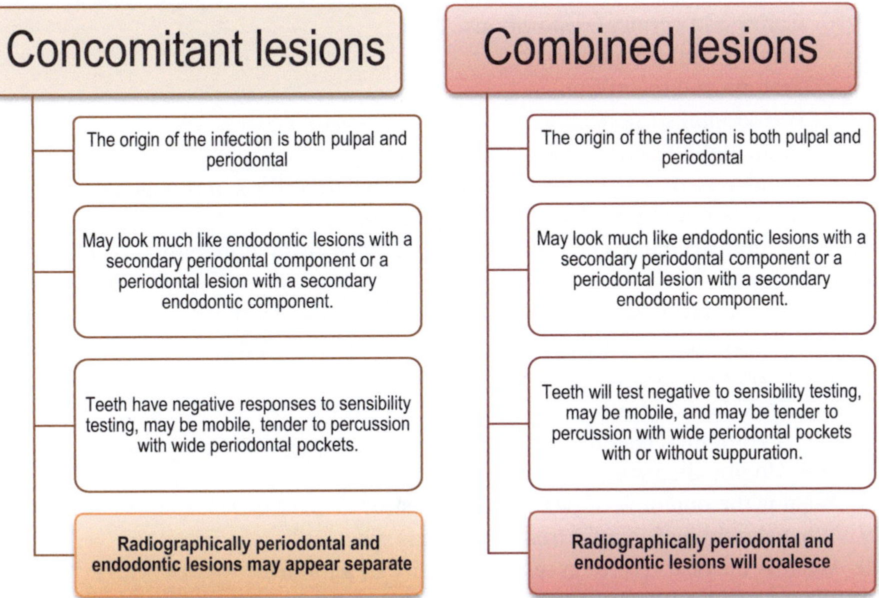

Fig. 10.3 Summary of the main learning points for teeth with true perio-endo lesions

Dento-Legal Aspects

In order for an informed decision to be made, especially with perio-endo lesions, it is imperative that the prognosis and options are discussed with the patient before embarking on treatment. The treatment outcomes can be unpredictable, and may not necessarily improve the longevity of the tooth enough to warrant the time and resources required for saving the tooth. The patient needs to be informed and understand the alternative options to treatment of the perio-endo involved tooth, as the potential prognosis and outcomes of the replacement options may be better in some circumstances.

Test Your Learning

Try to answer the following questions to test your learning:

1. Can you list the causes of communication between the periodontal tissues and the pulpal tissues?
2. Can you think of the process by which these insults affect the perio-endo interface?
      Caries and cervical restorations
      Scaling and root planing
      Trauma and resorption
      Periodontal surgery
      Endodontic treatment/surgery
3. Can you classify the various resorptive cases described in this book according to the Abbott and Lin Classification (2022)?
4. What improvement (in mm) do you expect from non-surgical periodontal treatment?
5. How can parafunction lead to the loss of vitality of teeth?
6. Can you summarise the clinical and radiographic findings for a lesion of
      (a) Periodontal origin
      (b) Endodontic origin
      (c) A combined lesion
7. How do you diagnose periodontal disease?
8. What is the outcome of periodontal disease?
9. What should periodontal treatment focus most on?
10. What is the best way to assess the vitality of a tooth?
11. What are the pathways for endodontic lesions to drain?
12. How do you diagnose a cracked tooth?
13. What leads to a successful outcome in root canal treatment and what are the expected outcomes of endodontic treatment?
14. What are the key features of perio-endo lesions?
15. How do you classify perio-endo lesions?
16. What treatment options are there for a true perio-endo lesion and what is the expected outcome?
17. What are the treatment options for an unsalvageable tooth?

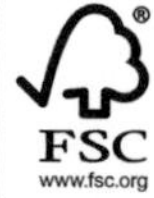

MIX
Papier aus verantwortungsvollen Quellen
Paper from responsible sources
FSC® C105338

If you have any concerns about our products,
you can contact us on
ProductSafety@springernature.com

In case Publisher is established outside the EU,
the EU authorized representative is:
Springer Nature Customer Service Center GmbH
Europaplatz 3, 69115 Heidelberg, Germany

Printed by Libri Plureos GmbH
in Hamburg, Germany